Specialist Training in
DERMATOLOGY

Edited by

Andrew Y. Finlay MBBS FRCP

Professor of Dermatology
Cardiff University
Cardiff, Wales, UK

Mahbub M. U. Chowdhury MBChB FRCP

Consultant in Occupational Dermatology
University Hospital of Wales
Cardiff, Wales, UK

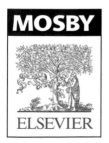

MOSBY

ELSEVIER

Edinburgh London New York Oxford Philadelphia St Louis Sydney Toronto 2007

MOSBY
ELSEVIER

An imprint of Elsevier Limited

First published 2007

ISBN 0 7234 3399 2
ISBN-13 978 0 7234 3399 6

British Library Cataloguing in Publication Data
A catalogue record for this book is available from the British Library

Library of Congress Cataloging in Publication Data
A catalog record for this book is available from the Library of Congress

Notice

Knowledge and best practice in this field are constantly changing. As new research and experience broaden our knowledge, changes in practice, treatment and drug therapy may become necessary or appropriate. Readers are advised to check the most current information provided (i) on procedures featured or (ii) by the manufacturer of each product to be administered, to verify the recommended dose or formula, the method and duration of administration, and contraindications. It is the responsibility of the practitioner, relying on their own experience and knowledge of the patient, to make diagnoses, to determine dosages and the best treatment for each individual patient, and to take all appropriate safety precautions. To the fullest extent of the law, neither the Publisher nor the Editors assume any liability for any injury and/or damage to persons or property arising out of or related to any use of the material contained in this book.

The Publisher

Working together to grow
libraries in developing countries

www.elsevier.com | www.bookaid.org | www.sabre.org

ELSEVIER   BOOK AID International   Sabre Foundation

ELSEVIER   your source for books, journals and multimedia in the health sciences
www.elsevierhealth.com

The publisher's policy is to use paper manufactured from sustainable forests

Printed in China

Contents

Contributors

Christian R. Aldridge BSc (Hons) MBBCh MRCP
Specialist Registrar in Dermatology
Glan Clwyd Hospital
Rhyl, Wales, UK

Alex V. Anstey MBBS DRCOG MD FRCP
Consultant Dermatologist &
Honorary Senior Lecturer
Royal Gwent Hospital
Newport, Wales, UK

Avinash S. Belgi MBBS MD MRCP
Specialist Registrar in Dermatology
University Hospital of Wales
Cardiff, Wales, UK

Sharon L. W. Blackford MBBCh FRCP
Consultant Dermatologist
Singleton Hospital
Swansea, Wales, UK

Mahbub M. U. Chowdhury MBChB FRCP
Consultant in Occupational Dermatology
University Hospital of Wales
Cardiff, Wales, UK

Andrew Y. Finlay MBBS FRCP
Professor of Dermatology
Cardiff University
Cardiff, Wales, UK

Peter J. A. Holt MBChB FRCP
Consultant Dermatologist
University Hospital of Wales
Cardiff, Wales, UK

Cherng Jong MBBS MRCP
Specialist Registrar in Dermatology
Singleton Hospital
Swansea, Wales, UK

Manjunatha Kalavala MBBS MD MRCP
Specialist Registrar in Dermatology
Singleton Hospital
Swansea, Wales, UK

Victoria J. Lewis BMedSci (Hons) MBBS MRCP
Specialist Registrar in Dermatology
University Hospital of Wales
Cardiff, Wales, UK

Richard A. Logan MBChB FRCP
Consultant Dermatologist
Princess of Wales Hospital
Bridgend, Wales, UK

Colin C. Long MBBS FRCP
Consultant Dermatologist
Llandough Hospital &
University Hospital of Wales
Cardiff, Wales, UK

Andrew D. Morris MBBCh MRCP
Consultant Dermatologist
University Hospital of Wales
Cardiff, Wales, UK

Richard J. Motley MBBChir MA MD FRCP
Consultant Dermatologist
University Hospital of Wales
Cardiff, Wales, UK

Nicolas G. Nicolaou MBBCh MRCP
Consultant Dermatologist
Royal Gwent Hospital
Newport, Wales, UK

Girish K. Patel MBBS MD MRCP
Formerly Specialist Registrar in
Dermatology
University Hospital of Wales
Cardiff, Wales, UK

Anthony D. Pearse MSc FIScT
Senior Research Fellow
Cardiff University
Cardiff, Wales, UK

Angela Steen RGN DipN Cert Ed
Clinical Nurse Specialist in Dermatology
Glan Clwyd Hospital
Rhyl, Wales, UK

Richard E. A. Williams BMedSci (Hons) BMBS
FRCP
Consultant Dermatologist
Glan Clwyd Hospital
Rhyl, Wales, UK

Diane J. Williamson MBChB FRCP
Consultant Dermatologist
Glan Clwyd Hospital
Rhyl, Wales, UK

Preface

There are plenty of excellent reference books to turn to when wanting more facts about a skin disease. This book seeks to meet a different need. When you start training in dermatology, how do you go about making sense of this completely new world of medicine? All those years of training in the broader aspects of internal medicine are essential to build on, but how can you rapidly progress to being able to function in a demanding training post?

This book is aimed at the novice in dermatology. The authors have all been involved either as trainees or trainers in the Specialist Registrar training scheme in Wales. This combination of experience and current insight into what a new Specialist Registrar really needs to know gives the pages direct relevance to many aspects of a trainee's day. The book is packed with practical tips including, for example, how to handle common clinical situations, how to begin to get into research or how to approach your surgical experience.

The key subjects from the UK and European curricula for dermatology training are introduced in the 13 chapters. Read early in training, many of the chapters will make the building up of much more detailed knowledge easier.

As well as being of interest to trainee dermatologists, we hope that this book will be of help to specialist dermatology nurses, general practitioners wanting to develop their practical understanding of the subject, and to medical students or junior doctors considering the possibility of dermatology as a career. We would welcome any suggestions and corrections for future editions.

Andrew Y. Finlay
Mahbub M. U. Chowdhury

Foreword

Skin disease is very common; it is estimated that at any one time approximately 50% of the population has a dermatosis of one kind or another and 25% of them would benefit from medical attention. If there were to be proportional representation of prevalence of diseases of any one organ and the number of trainees in the specialty dealing with those diseases then dermatology would be the best represented. Sadly this is not the case. A working knowledge of dermatology is of help to any clinician from surgeon to psychiatrist; dermatologists are most probably consulted more frequently by their colleagues than any other specialist.

On the face of it dermatology appears 'easy'; as it is visual and accessible everyone believes they can diagnose 'simple' skin diseases such as acne or psoriasis and most times they can. However, and paradoxically, the specialty is highly complex and diagnosis is fraught with pitfalls; the number of diagnoses — 2000 — bears testimony to this. Frequently a diagnosis is arrived at as a result of close consultation between pathologist and experienced clinician mainly because histology is not always pathognomonic. Dermatology is probably the last of the true clinical specialties being reliant on the clinician's skills and experience with relatively little recourse to instrumentation. As in other branches of medicine dermatologists are busy subspecializing. Consultants may choose to specialize in a variety of areas including academia, photobiology, dermatological surgery, medical dermatology, paediatric dermatology, contact dermatitis, immuno-bullous diseases, vulval disease, etc. In short there is something for everyone whether they be surgically or medically inclined.

A recent survey of senior medical students in the USA revealed that the number ranking dermatology as their first choice career option had increased ten-fold over the past decade. The reason behind this is quite simple — dermatology offers a controllable lifestyle, so important and desirable nowadays. This is mirrored in the UK; entrance to specialist registrar training programmes in dermatology is fiercely competitive. Despite this interest trainees in dermatology are faced with a conundrum in that the teaching of dermatology in British medical schools has declined significantly at the same time as applications to train in the specialty has reached an all-time high. Although most first year specialist registrars will have been a senior house officer, Foundation Year 2 or locum appointment in dermatology before gaining a training number their knowledge of dermatology will be rudimentary. Indeed the dermatological lexicon is alien to most young doctors. The descriptive terminologies for skin lesions such as 'macule' or 'vesicle' and the names of diseases such as pityriasis rubra pilaris, etc. are not learnt in medical school. The structured

4-year training programme in dermatology in the UK is short and intense and no longer the leisurely apprenticeship of old. Learning the basics of the discipline are important, particularly as opportunities for hands-on training are encroached upon by assessment in competency and knowledge. Before setting out into the relative unknown it would be useful for the aspiring dermatologist to have a travel guide to dermatology to allow him, or increasingly her, to plan the journey and stay on track.

The guide edited by Finlay and Chowdhury with their colleagues from the Welsh dermatology training programme is just such a travelogue. The all-important chapters on diagnosis and management of skin disease are there, as they would be in any textbook on dermatology. However, what sets this text apart is the in-depth coverage of those areas that one would wish to know at the beginning of training rather than halfway through or even at the end—the areas that should be taught but so often aren't because they are not 'ticks' on the curriculum, for instance descriptions of the myriad of dermatological subspecialties, advice on management and how to deal with hospital managers and the practicalities of running an outpatient service. Particularly important is the central, literally up front, role that academics and research are given with sound practical advice as to how to get started in research, what career options are open to the aspiring academic, how to apply for research funding and of course how to get the resultant work published.

Although not a substitute for a dermatological major reference book this book is exactly what a new trainee would wish to have close at hand to guide them to the opportunities and around the pitfalls awaiting them in their chosen career.

Christopher E. M. Griffiths
Professor of Dermatology
The University of Manchester
Manchester, UK

Acknowledgements

Dr Logan is grateful to Dr Margaret Cotter and Dr Jim Neal for their help in preparing the photomicrographs in Chapter 3, and also to the staff of the Histopathology Laboratory at the Princess of Wales Hospital for their patience.

Ms Angela Steen and Dr Williamson would like to thank Mr Mike Jones, Medical Photographer, Conwy & Denbighshire NHS Trust for his help and co-operation with Chapter 9.

The Editors would like to thank Mrs Susan Williams for her secretarial assistance, and the staff of the Department of Media Resources, University Hospital of Wales for their contribution and help.

Conflict of interest: Professor A. Y. Finlay is joint copyright owner of the Dermatology Life Quality Index (DLQI), Psoriasis Disability Index (PDI) and the Children's Dermatology Life Quality Index (CDQI).

Research and write

1

Girish K. Patel and Andrew Y. Finlay

INTRODUCTION

All dermatology trainees should be given the opportunity to participate in research. But why undertake research? When is it best to start a project and what type of project should you choose? In this chapter we address these age-old questions and offer advice on how to make your research endeavours successful.

WHY UNDERTAKE RESEARCH?

Believe it or not, by choosing to be a dermatologist you have chosen a dynamic research-led specialty. Most dermatologists in the UK have published. Skin-related research leads the way in many spheres of scientific endeavour and patient care.

Research is the practice of finding more about the world around us, so that understanding can be used to better manage it. Everyday we explore, generate and test hypotheses, in order to make conclusions; we are in fact carrying out research. Much meaningful research has been conducted in big laboratories, usually in pharmaceutical companies or big government funded institutions. But today dermatology research is conducted the world over, the technical skills are readily transferable and the only constraint is imagination. Small focused laboratories are now able to make big scientific strides on the back of readily available amassed information.

The demands on a specialist registrar are well known, but can be overcome. Undertake research when you are ready and only undertake research you are interested in. In keeping with Murphy's law: if there is a chance that things can go wrong they invariably do and the only driving force to complete a project will be your desire to succeed. Supervisors look foremost for motivated individuals, as technical skills can be taught but not motivation. Research success comes from a motivated person working in a supportive environment.

WHEN SHOULD I DO RESEARCH?

As a senior house officer or a specialist registrar in dermatology your immediate priority is to establish safe and efficient clinical competences. But make use of the time allotted for research. Of course with time if your interest in research grows you will naturally look to expand your research sessions. You might be able to free up additional sessions by cross covering with colleagues, who are also trying to free up additional time. Start on a small project that you can complete within months. You will be surprised at how long it takes to complete a project and publish. When you enter a new post try to find a simple case report based on a startling observation. Make sure the patient has provided written consent for clinical photographs to be used for medical publication. Then take care to write it up promptly and see it through to publication; this is often the first rung of the ladder.

WHAT TYPE OF RESEARCH SHOULD I CONDUCT?

Over the last two decades the NHS has adopted a number of initiatives to improve the quality of clinical practice. Two of these approaches have stood the test of time: evidence-based medicine (EBM) and clinical audit. EBM is associated with the production of clinical protocols, guidelines and standards, which can be re-engineered to produce clinical care pathways. Clinical audit on the other hand is used to evaluate and improve implementation of such pathways. These approaches now form the foundation for improving healthcare delivery, as well as facilitating policy decision-making and resource allocation.

Clinical audit

During your training you will be required to undertake clinical audit. Begin by identifying an area of clinical practice that is amenable to improvement; there are many examples (Table 1.1).

The first step in undertaking an audit is to identify all the key components of the process, from beginning to end (Figure 1.1).

Then define a standard(s) that you can measure for each component and the acceptable benchmark for this standard that will demonstrate efficiency at that step. This standard needs to be clearly defined so that data collection is free of ambiguity. Poorly defined standards are the major cause of failure of implementation of audit changes.

Next choose one component of the process pathway that you believe will yield most to a simple intervention and undertake a comprehensive survey to verify this and measure the standard for this step. It is important that this is a comprehensive survey that includes all variables. This is much more important than trying to survey an entire process. After collating and analysing the data you should be able to present your findings and clearly state how far short the current practice falls from the acceptable benchmark, as well as making a credible case for an intervention.

Table 1.1

Clinical audit categories	Example of such a process	An example of a standard and benchmark	Example of an initiative that may improve the process
Contractual requirements for service delivery	Number of outpatients seen	No patient non-attendance	Patient initiated telephone verification of appointment
Training	Research time	3 hour bleep free time per week	Internal cover timetable
Patient care	Inpatients' satisfaction	All patients should know their named nurse	Create an inpatient information pack
Care pathway protocols	Surgical procedures	Every patient should sign a consent form	Make available consent forms in outpatients prior to booking the procedure
Drug safety	Prescription of azathioprine	Every patient should have a thiopurine-methyl-transferase assay	Make available a drug checklist and monitoring sheet that can be incorporated into the medical notes
Local protocols such as shared care	Methotrexate prescribing	No interruption in treatment or its monitoring	Make available patient held drug monitoring cards and clear protocols of care
Professional body (BAD) guidelines	Treatment of non-melanoma skin cancer	Appropriate surgical margins for excision	Make a template for documentation of each tumour type
National professional body (RCP) guidelines	Osteoporosis	DEXA scan for all patients under 60 years of age prescribed corticosteroids	Clear lines of collaboration with DEXA service
National (NICE) guidelines	Appropriate use of biologics	Patients should meet criteria for receiving such medication	Criteria made available to all care givers
Health costs	Isotretinoin prescribing	No patient should require the more expensive 5mg tablet	Restrict prescription of the 5mg dose from pharmacy

However, to complete the audit cycle you will be expected to implement your change and repeat the survey. There is a highly recommended guide to clinical audit written by Professor Gawkrodger on behalf of the British Association of Dermatologists.[1]

Good quality audit projects can often be published, either as an abstract submitted to a national or international meeting or as a short article. You should aim to carry out any audit to a standard that would potentially make it publishable if successful.

Medical research

A clear distinction is made in medical research between laboratory-based research, 'at the bench', and clinical research, 'at the bedside'. As practising clinicians there is a clear bias towards clinical research. All trainees should dip their toe in the water and carry out at

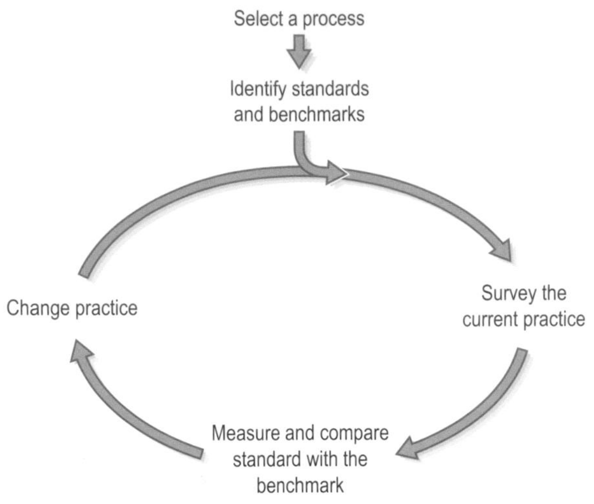

Figure 1.1
Clinical audit.

Select a process

Identify standards
and benchmarks

Change practice

Survey the
current practice

Measure and compare
standard with the
benchmark

least one clinical trial. A Specialist Registrar (SpR), by the end of their training, should be comfortable formulating a clinical project and taking it through to completion. In the past dermatologists had been trained to appreciate both clinical and laboratory research. However, the transit time in the current SpR programme is often seen as a barrier to such luxuries. Today the boundaries between these two approaches are diminishing due to the increased emphasis on translational research. The new model for successful research is to ensure that observations made at the bedside are rapidly addressed at the bench and new diagnostic tools or therapies developed, which can then be evaluated once more at the bedside.

WHERE DO I START AND WHAT ARE THE HURDLES?

Finding the hypothesis

All good research should start with a question, which can then be pared down further to a yes/no answer. This then is the basis of a hypothesis, a question that can be tested. Herein lies one of the great paradigms of modern research, that it is easier to refute a hypothesis than to prove it, thus favouring a reductionist approach.

Literature search and critical appraisal

Has anyone else thought of trying to test your hypothesis? If so what approach did they use? To answer these questions you need to conduct a literature search. This involves four main challenges:

- deciding where to search;
- using the defined research question (the hypothesis) to devise a search strategy;
- critically appraising the information collected; and
- storing references for easy access.

Searching PubMed, with or without Boolean search operations, is a minimum requirement. Limit your search by subheadings (e.g. aetiology, treatment ...) or language, age group or publication year. There are numerous other electronic science search engines that may be more appropriate and include: Google Scholar, OVID, Web of science, Cochrane database, Embase. And of course use a conventional search engine such as Google; to avoid junk use phrases in inverted commas and carefully look at the URLs (Table 1.2).

Don't forget the old fashioned ways that still work; the use of an up-to-date textbook, review articles and most importantly cross-referencing (looking up the references of an article). A clear search strategy helps to refine and update your search at a later stage.

The hardest part of the process is to prioritize and carefully go through all the papers. Critical appraisal is a way to rationalize the amassed papers. Some basic questions to always ask yourself are listed in Table 1.3, and for further guidance read the papers by Trisha Greenhalgh in the BMJ on how to read a paper.[2–11]

WRITING A PROTOCOL

Even the simplest clinical study needs a clear detailed written protocol before starting. This is essential for ethical review, for institutional permission and for financial planning.

Table 1.2: URLs

.ac	Academic
.edu	US university
.gov	Government site
.org	Not for profit organization
.com or .co	Company

Table 1.3: Critical appraisal

	Yes	No
Do I know the research group and can you trust it?		
Is there a relevant question?		
Is it clearly focused, in terms of the population, methods and outcomes?		
Are these the best/correct methods to answer the question?		
Is the population studied correct and accounted for?		
How did they randomize and blind their intervention?		
Are compared groups similar?		
Apart from the intervention, were both groups treated the same?		
How large was the effect?		
Did they consider confounding and bias?		
Was the follow-up long enough?		
Are the data shown clearly interpretable?		
Are the statistics okay?		
Who funded the study?		
Is it applicable locally?		

However, equally importantly, the intellectual process of thinking about and writing the protocol is the essential basis for ensuring that the work is successful.

How to start

Protocol housekeeping

The protocol will go through several versions before it is ready to submit for review. First write the date and the draft number 1! Update this heading for each version. Without this basic information you and co-workers will become irritatingly confused by different versions.

Title of study

Choose a clear descriptive and preferably interesting study title. Remember that you need to enthuse your co-workers and to interest the various committee members who will have to review your protocol.

Researchers involved

Decide who you want involved, get their agreement and list their names. This list defines who you can expect to (and by default who will not) contribute. It also defines who will expect to be authors on eventual abstracts or publications.

Background

Two or three paragraphs of background are essential. The writing of this forces clarification of the reasoning behind the study. This information is important to convince the ethical committee and other review committees that the work is worth doing. The background should be referenced, including the most relevant recent references to the proposed work. The background should clarify how the current published work has led to a certain level of understanding about the subject, and should clarify how the proposed study leads logically forward addressing currently unanswered questions. The work in writing the protocol background is not 'wasted' as it can be used later as the basis of the introduction paragraphs of the manuscript for publication based on the study.

Decide the aims

It is essential to write down a clear aim of any proposed study. Identify as few aims as possible, preferably only one. If you try to answer one question, you may succeed. If you try to answer five questions, you will fail. State the main aim and the question to be answered. Document any subsidiary aim.

Method (study design)

In writing the methods section, you should plan to give enough detail so that the study could be carried out successfully even if you were not able to have any input. Think through the reality of the study, imagining every step, anticipating questions that may arise and writing down the instructions.

Clarify whether the study is an open study, controlled, single or double blinded.

Patient selection

Define the entry criteria, e.g. define the disease or level of activity of disease for entry, sex and age range. Define exclusion criteria, such as pregnancy or presence of other diseases. Decide the number of patients to be studied. The advice of a statistician is important at this stage. Clarify how and where recruitment is to take place. Where are patients going to be found? In deciding this be very aware of the potential for selection bias influencing the outcome of the study.

Controls

If the study is planned to include controls, they need to be defined with as much care as for patients. Decide on entry and exclusion criteria. State how the controls are to be matched to the patients, and how they are to be recruited.

Intervention

If a treatment or other intervention is being tested, this needs to be clearly defined. If a drug is being studied, the dosage and frequency need to be stated. If the drug is topical, clear definitions should be given of how much is to be applied, and to where. Consider any techniques to be used to monitor compliance, such as patient diaries or weighing application containers.

Assessment criteria

It is essential to decide on the ways that are to be used to measure the effects of the proposed intervention. These should be clearly defined, e.g. use of SCORAD in a study on atopic dermatitis. The chosen techniques should be as simple as possible, and consideration should be given to defining reproducibility between observers if, in the study, more than one observer is to be involved. Consider if there are objective methods available to use as outcome measures, e.g. ultrasound to measure psoriasis plaque thickness.

Patient information sheet

The patient information sheet is an integral part of any protocol. Write in simple English, using straightforward non-technical terms. Be honest. Use clear paragraph headings such as 'What have I to do?' or 'Are there any possible side effects?'. Give contact names and phone numbers, and give indemnity details.

Patient consent form

This is an integral part of the protocol. You will need to adhere to local institutional guidelines and national requirements.

Statistician

It is important to discuss the proposed protocol with a statistician before submitting the study for ethical review. Advice on number of patients, data collection and design is helpful at this stage. It is no good going to a statistician after a study has been completed, seeking help on the interpretation of data, and discovering that fundamental avoidable mistakes have been made.

Costing

All studies use resources. These resources need to be costed and decisions need to be taken about who will pay. Remember in costing studies that realistic estimates need to be taken about how much time you and your co-workers will spend on the study. Remember secretarial time, nursing time and patient expenses. This is discussed further in the Seeking funding section below.

Indemnity

It is essential to clarify the indemnity arrangement for any study involving patients or other volunteers. Indemnity may be provided by an NHS trust, by a university and/or by a pharmaceutical company. Personal insurance cover is also essential. Advice should be sought about these matters.

Ethical approval

Any study involving patients or volunteers must be approved by the appropriate ethical committee before starting a study. Indemnity cover will almost certainly be invalid until approval in writing is received.

Seeking funding

A major challenge for UK academic dermatologists is finding funding; for some it is a career-long quest. Funds from the government, in the form of a Medical Research Council (MRC, http://www.mrc.ac.uk) award are unfortunately in short supply, most of us rely heavily upon charitable donations — see Box 1.1. What is more controversial is funding received from undertaking clinical trials for pharmaceutical companies; 'soft monies'. This is especially the case if your project involves a product from one of these companies, for it is often difficult to shake off the perception of study bias. The bottom line is that it is not possible to undertake research without funding.

Herein lies a major challenge: without a proven track record of academic achievement it is often not possible to get funding, without which it is impossible to undertake research to build up an academic profile. A hot tip: as soon as possible identify a senior staff member capable of getting research funding and ask for their advice. At the same time start by applying for travel fellowships at the British Association of Dermatologists/Dowling Club to build up a track record of winning and securing funds. Those who have decided on an academic career could consider the trainee fellowships offered by the MRC or Wellcome Trust.

Box 1.1: Sources of research funding

- Medical Research Council (MRC, http://www.mrc.ac.uk)
- Wellcome Trust (http://www.wellcome.ac.uk)
- Cancer Research UK (http://www.cancerresearchuk.org)
- British Skin Foundation (BSF, http://www.britishskinfoundation.org.uk)
- Dystrophic Epidermolysis Bullosa Charity (DebRA, http://debra.org)
- Psoriasis Association (http://www.psoriasis-association.org.uk/)
- National Eczema Society (htpp://www.eczema.org/)

THE PATH TO SUCCESSFUL RESEARCH

Saying 'NO'

For some this represents the biggest barrier to success. When undertaking research, especially in the laboratory, interruptions such as those from bleeps can have detrimental consequences. Due to the limited availability of time it is not possible to complete all the tasks asked of you. Hence you have to be able to prioritize and develop the ability to say NO with sincerity and diplomacy, within the limits of your employment contract.

Pick and choose your projects carefully. Choose projects that you can see being completed in a practical timeframe. Stagger projects, so that at any one time you are not writing up two projects simultaneously. Plan some slack into your schedule, because in clinical practice the unexpected and delays are the norm.

The mentor

We all need mentors to guide us through difficult career decisions. Choose your mentor carefully. A good mentor will listen and understand the issues that concern you. Most importantly they will give you advice that you can trust even when it is unfavourable. Great mentors are unfortunately few, but when you find one their effervescence can brighten up the most sullied day.

Clear questions, ideal methods and data analysis

Choosing the correct research question to answer is the most important factor in defining the success of a project. The best scientific papers resolve hypotheses that are understood by all and thus their relevance is far reaching. The ability to identify such opportunities comes from an in-depth understanding of the subject area, experience and a creative intellect. Many investigators will spend a month or more discussing the project area with their student, working through the merits of a variety of approaches to tackle the research opportunity. After this point it is difficult to go back. Though you should always strive to use the best methodological approach to address the hypothesis, this has to balanced against the time it takes to derive results. Remember that the research field is competitive and the rewards are less for those that come second. Statistical analysis provides confidence against a chance finding. There are many statistical approaches and although you should have a basic idea of statistical techniques, it is prudent to consult with a statistician *before* carrying out a project. A statistician can help you calculate the number of subjects required for a study to derive a meaningful result. If a study requires a lot of subjects, then consider a pilot study to test the methodology beforehand.

'Publish or perish'

A clear measure of success is the ability to publish, hence the phrase 'publish or perish'. Publications can take the form of an abstract, case-report, basic science or clinical trial paper, review article or book chapter. For some writing comes naturally, though for most of us it is a skill that we acquire by practice. Choose the journal to publish in carefully. A good measure of the strength of a journal is the number of times articles within it are cited. The impact factor published by the Thomson Institute for Scientific Information (http://www.sciencegateway.org/impact/) is also used when measuring the success of an academic department (Box 1.2 — most recent figures are for 2005).

The pathway to publication is often fraught with traps and delays, but stick at it and you will prevail; this is particularly true for your first publication. The process takes much longer than may seem possible (Figure 1.2).

HOW TO WRITE THE FIRST DRAFT OF YOUR ARTICLE

The most common reason that clinical research studies are not published is that they are never submitted for publication. This is how to avoid that depressing outcome.

First, immediately a study is completed, sit down and start writing. If you have not written an article based on a clinical research study before, you may need help in overcoming the 'how do I start?' confusion that you may initially feel. In fact it is not as difficult as it seems.

Write '1st draft. Date. Your name'. On the next line give the title of the paper. Next write the names of all the authors, with your name first. Then give the institution(s) that employ the authors. Next write your contact address, telephone and fax numbers and email address for correspondence. The first heading is Abstract or Summary. After this leave a

Box 1.2

Scientific journals	Impact factor
Science	30.9
Cell	29.4
Nature	29.3
Nature Medicine	28.9
Journal of Clinical Investigation	15.1
Journal of Experimental Medicine	14.0

Medical journals	
New England Journal of Medicine	44.0
Lancet	23.4
Journal of the American Medical Association	23.3
Annals of Internal Medicine	13.3
British Medical Journal	9.1

Dermatology journals	
Journal of Investigative Dermatology	4.4
Archives of Dermatology	3.4
British Journal of Dermatology	3.0
Journal of the American Academy of Dermatology	2.4
Dermatological Surgery	2.3

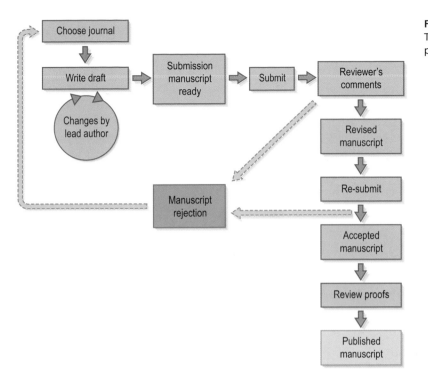

Figure 1.2
The process of publication.

blank for the time being; this can be completed later. The next heading is Introduction. You wrote this some time ago as the background paragraphs for the protocol. Cut and paste it across: there may need to be some minor adjustments, for example in the tenses used.

The next heading is Methods. Again, all of the details are already in the protocol, so this can also be copied and minor changes made. The Results heading is next. Start to write this as completely as possible, leaving many blanks where the data have not yet been analysed. Having this template makes the process of data analysis more focused. The next heading is Discussion. You can usually write at least half of this without the final results being ready. This is where you can raise issues, difficulties or perceived weaknesses of the study — better to point these out rather than having the manuscript turned down. The results should be placed in context with other previously published work, some of which may have been referred to in the introduction.

The next heading is Acknowledgements. Here you can thank those who have contributed but whose contributions were not sufficient to warrant authorship. You can also thank patients or doctors who helped recruit subjects. Funding can be acknowledged here. Remember to list any conflict of interest either here or in the covering letter to the editor when the manuscript is submitted.

The list of References should be added to, accurately in Vancouver style (as used by the British Journal of Dermatology and most major medical journals), each time you mention a reference in the text. It is usually better at draft stage to list the reference in the text thus: 'Brown and Green, 2006' and only substitute a superscript number at the last draft before submission.

Tables and Figures should be listed, along with the descriptor for each. Following this each Table and Figure should be given on a separate page (Table 1.4).

After completing the above, you are already half way there, and most importantly you have got a first draft, which must now be reviewed and amended by the co-authors. Decide which journal you are going to first submit the article to and read the instructions for authors for that journal. Reformat the manuscript as necessary. Now you should evaluate the data with a statistician. Put the results into a second draft and circulate it to all planned co-authors. Redraft, rewrite, redraft, rewrite. Do not expect too much input from your co-authors, it is human nature to let the main author bear most of the burden of the work. Do not let non-contributing authors hold things up. If you get no response politely give deadlines, stating you will continue anyway if they are not met. Finally, do not rest until the manuscript has finally been submitted for publication. The process of preparing the manuscript can often take discouraging turns, for which you must be resilient. You must expect either to be asked to make various changes or to have the manuscript rejected. If asked to make changes, go to considerable trouble to answer and to try to meet every suggestion — this is the best way to ensure eventual acceptance.[12] If the manuscript is rejected, again make changes based on the referee's comments but do not give up; identify another journal and resubmit.

FULLTIME RESEARCH AND HIGHER DEGREES

If after a period of time you find the challenge of research enticing, the time restraints imposed by clinical training become burdensome. A practical approach to this problem is

Table 1.4: Layout for first draft	
Title page	Write draft number, date and your name Title List of authors, institutions Correspondence details
Introduction	This should be a broad description leading to the question your study addresses Mostly derived from the protocol
Methods	Mostly derived from the protocol
Results	Give a detailed summary of all the findings in a logical order
Discussion	This should put your study findings into the context of the known literature Discuss perceived difficulties, weaknesses and strengths of your study
Acknowledgements	Thank contributions from those not sufficient to warrant authorship Funding sources Conflicts of interest statement
References	Begin with the Vancouver style, though this may change depending on the journal you wish to submit to
Legends	Should clearly describe the data presented in the figures
Figures and tables	These should be stand alone data, easily interpreted with the help of the legend

to devote a period of your career to fulltime research. Such positions are often sought after and usually mean a drop in salary unless they are linked to clinical tasks. By committing to such a career change you must seriously consider the merits of completing a higher degree, be that an MD or PhD. In addition to providing a full on experience of research, for further academic endeavour a higher degree is a prerequisite.

The difference between an MD and PhD has become obscure over time. In the past the MD was regarded as a more clinical degree in which the project was initiated and carried out by the student, taking anywhere between 2 and 4 years fulltime. For a PhD the project is often chosen by the supervisor, it is primarily based at the laboratory bench and is conducted over 4 to 6 years. The boundary between the two types of degree is now blurred. A more telling factor is often the ability to retain a National Training Number for the time away from direct patient care, without which of course training as a dermatologist cannot be completed. In most instances, postgraduate deans are happy to allow up to one year of training to be utilized for such academic endeavours.

FELLOWSHIPS AND RESEARCH ABROAD

For most individuals bitten by the research bug, completing a higher degree only reinforces the need to apply for a substantive post-doctoral position in order to master the skills necessary to conduct independent research. This has major implications for clinical skills and of course revalidation. In the current climate such a position should only be entertained after completion of specialist training, as this allows greater flexibility when returning. However, some individuals do leave their training number behind and risk re-applying for training positions upon their return to clinical work. Other issues, such as funding (usually in the form of fellowships), the project and location come into play. Many individuals, rightly or wrongly, believe that such a post should be abroad and among the favourites is the United States of America. Though many places in the USA will be happy to fund you as a Post-Doctorate Fellow, to maintain one's clinical income is more difficult and most UK based funding organisations appear reluctant to fund researchers going abroad. With the opening of European borders the situation may be different for positions within the European Union.

BUT IN THE END …

Whether or not you decide to pursue your academic endeavours to post-doctoral level or beyond, at the heart of dermatology there remains a desire to maintain research. There is a common misconception that interest in research is only for those pursuing the ever-perilous journey up the university hierarchy. Nothing could be further from the truth; all forms of research can be continued whilst in a consultant post and there are many such successful examples in the UK. It is important to realize that research in its various forms offers a mind-set that questions and allows one to answer the uncertainties that surround us in daily practice. By participating you will enrich your own career, as well as impact directly on the future wellbeing of patients.

References

1. Gawkrodger DJ. Medical audit for dermatologists a practical guide. London: British Association of Dermatologists; 1994.
2. Greenhalgh T. How to read a paper. The Medline database. BMJ 1997; 315:180–183.
3. Greenhalgh T. How to read a paper. Getting your bearings (deciding what the paper is about). BMJ 1997; 315:243–246.
4. Greenhalgh T. How to read a paper. Assessing the methodological quality of published papers. BMJ 1997; 315:305–308.
5. Greenhalgh T. How to read a paper. Statistics for the non-statistician. I: different types of data need different statistical tests. BMJ 1997; 315:364–366.
6. Greenhalgh T. How to read a paper. Statistics for the non-statistician. II: 'Significant' relations and their pitfalls. BMJ 1997; 315:422–425.
7. Greenhalgh T. How to read a paper. Papers that report drug trials. BMJ 1997; 315:480–483.
8. Greenhalgh T. How to read a paper. Papers that report diagnostic or screening tests. BMJ 1997; 315:540–543.
9. Greenhalgh T. How to read a paper. Papers that tell you what things cost (economic analyses). BMJ 1997; 315:596–599.
10. Greenhalgh T. How to read a paper. Papers that summarize other papers (systematic reviews and meta-analyses). BMJ 1997; 315:672–675.
11. Greenhalgh T. How to read a paper. Papers that go beyond numbers (qualitative research). BMJ 1997; 315:740–743.
12. Williams H. How to reply to referees. J Am Acad Dermatol 2004; 51:79–83.

Practical management skills

2

Christian R. Aldridge and Mahbub M. U. Chowdhury

INTRODUCTION

The title of this chapter may be reason enough to bypass this section of the book!

Before you move on to the 'interesting' bits take a few minutes to read this fictional account below of a possible interaction between senior and junior colleagues. Its themes will be expanded on later in the chapter.

> He knocked gently.
> 'Come in, come in.'
> The voice was assured and direct. The new registrar opened the door and was greeted effusively by a mass of pin-stripe.
> 'Fabulous to see you again,' he boomed, whilst pumping his hand. 'Hope you're ready for some hard work!'
> The registrar smiled nervously. He could feel the moisture collect in his palms. Just 8 weeks previously he had been a senior house officer, part of a successful dermatology team. Now, the reality of his appointment was beginning to seep through his shirt.
> 'Let's run through some ground rules, shall we?'
> The consultant pulled a small black chair from under his table and beckoned the registrar to sit.
> 'Now …, somewhere here I've got your time-table …'
> Looking over his spectacles, he was scanning the desk, his large, cuff-linked hand snaking its way through the piles of documents.
> 'It's never where you put it, is it?'
> He turned and raised his eyebrows at his junior.
> 'No, never,' he replied in a whisper.
> The consultant continued with his search.
> 'I'm sure I saw it … ah, here we go.'
> The consultant then leaned back in his chair, his waistcoat taking the strain of the numerous pharmaceutical dinners.
> 'Now, as you can see, you'll be doing four clinics a week with me and an extra peripheral clinic, which is not on your time-table, twice a month … on a Thursday …'
> His flow was interrupted by a phone call.
> 'Yes …, yes he's here with me now.'
> He cupped the receiver and mouthed 'My secretary'.
> 'A and E you say … hmm, I see … well … yes, I think that will be possible … I will tell him, thank you.'
> He replaced the handset and shrugged his shoulders.

'Looks like we've got a referral from A and E already … would you mind terribly seeing the patient after this meeting? It shouldn't take too long.'

The registrar shifted in his seat. The small polyester fibres from his seat were worming their way through his trousers, and beginning to sting.

'Yes, that's no problem,' he replied uneasily.

'Excellent, excellent … have you done any surgery?'

'A little bit but …'

'Excellent … you'll be having a list on a Monday. Small stuff really … few flaps and maybe the odd graft.'

The consultant rested his hand on his junior's shoulder.

'Shouldn't be a problem for someone as capable as you.'

The hand felt weighty, and he could definitely feel a squeeze too.

'Well, I guess it would be OK if there was some supervision …'

The registrar was interrupted by a knock on the door.

'Come in,' sighed the consultant.

It was the SHO.

'I've got the ward referrals you asked me to bring.'

She looks keen, thought the registrar, just like I was.

'Splendid … here you go, have a look at these and see what you think … is that OK?'

He handed over six, illegible pieces of paper. The registrar nodded feebly and stuffed them into his pocket. The SHO left and the consultant picked up his tan-coloured briefcase and thrust it into the registrar's hand.

'Walk with me.'

They marched out of the office down the three flights of stairs into the basement car-park, and walked up to the silver Mercedes parked in the corner. The leather briefcase was beginning to feel heavy by now.

'Right … I'll take that.'

The consultant popped open the boot and placed his bag inside. There was a large case of Bollinger champagne taking up most of the space.

'Daughter's wedding coming up,' he volunteered, as he shut the boot.

'I'm off to attend to a few things … can I leave you to supervise the team?'

The registrar's face began to sag. He could feel his jaw succumbing to gravity.

'There's a group of medical students that need a couple of tutorials today sometime … nothing too technical, though.'

The consultant tapped his junior's back reassuringly. The registrar stood dumbfounded as he watched the car drive out of the parking. Day one as a specialist registrar, he thought. Nice one.

This small excerpt was intended to give a flavour of the types of tasks a newly appointed specialist registrar may be asked to undertake. The purpose of this chapter is to highlight the important aspects of inpatient and outpatient management, on-call activity, ward referrals, primary healthcare and management skills.

OUTPATIENTS

Dermatology is essentially an outpatient based specialty. As a specialist registrar, you may see up to 1000 patients a year. The clinics are usually busy, to try to accommodate the increasing rate of referrals from general practitioners. This is not intended to reflect badly on general practitioners but demonstrates the gross under-representation of dermatology in the undergraduate and postgraduate curriculums.

The Joint Committee for Higher Medical Training (JCHMT) recommends that during the first year the trainee must do at least three general dermatology outpatient clinics per week. For at least 2 of the remaining 3 years, the trainee must do a minimum of three general dermatology clinics weekly. They advise that trainees should see both new and review patients. Thus, the aims within the 4-year training programme are to gain a fundamental understanding of general dermatology and to embellish this with specific sub-specialty learning as outlined in the working syllabus, provided by the JCHMT and also known as the logbook. It is vital to maintain an up-to-date record of your activities (Box 2.1).

Box 2.2 lists some useful tips on managing your outpatient clinic. Being punctual is extremely important and ensures a smooth start to the clinics. It is very difficult to catch up if one starts even a half hour late. This may sound obvious but has been shown to be one of the main reasons for clinics running behind schedule. One of the most taxing dichotomies in outpatient clinics for a specialist registrar is whether or not to ask for assistance. Do you check every patient with the consultant and risk them thinking that your patient management skills are poor or do you hold back in case the clinic begins to overrun? In reality, the majority of consultants are happy to discuss any issues you have about patient care. With time and experience comes confidence and the rate of consultation with the consultant will naturally fall. Most departments in the NHS now require at least 6 weeks' notice for annual and study leave so such requests must be made with good planning and all relevant personnel must be informed.

Box 2.1: *Maintaining a logbook*

- Earlier the better — record information while it is still fresh
- Stick to a routine — update your logbook at a set time
- Incomplete logbooks are useless
- Analyse regularly
- Use technology
- Ensure educational supervisor reports are up to date

Box 2.2: *Managing your outpatient clinic*

- Know exactly when and which clinics you are expected to attend
- Be punctual and arrive on time
- Inform your consultant if you will not be available for a clinic with good notice
- Decide whether you will dictate letters after seeing each patient (preferable) or whether you do all of them at the end of clinic
- Establish with your consultant when it is best to discuss patients
- Determine whether biopsies are performed within clinic times or on a designated biopsy list
- Get to know the outpatient nurses

ON CALL

The JCHMT stipulates, at present, that all trainees must have a non-resident on call commitment for dermatology for at least three out of four years of higher medical training. They recommend that the frequency of on call should not be less than a 1 in 7 rota and should cover the care of dermatology inpatients, handling ward referrals and general practitioner referrals and providing cover for the intensive care unit and the Accident and Emergency Department.

At present, no dermatology specialist registrar training programmes offer dual accreditation with general internal medicine. Therefore, it is not considered appropriate that trainees take part in on-call rotas for acute general medical emergencies. In fact, throughout many dermatology departments in the UK there have already been modifications to the on-call rotas for dermatology specialist registrars. Indeed, many units have phased out the 5 p.m.–9 a.m. on-call commitment, as this has traditionally been a relatively quiet time for referrals.

These changes have been forced onto the directorates following the implementation of the European Working Time Directive (EWTD) (Box 2.3) and the Hospital at Night Scheme (Box 2.4), which itself has been part of the NHS Modernisation Agency's Project to redefine how medical cover is provided in hospitals during the out of hours period.

Despite these changes, the bulk of dermatology referrals occur during daytime hours and it is still important to remain aware of best practice with regards to on-call cover (Box 2.5). Good communication is needed for on-call swaps: switchboard, wards, colleagues and secretaries should all be informed. When on call as non-resident doctors, it is particularly essential to be contactable at all times. You can be sure that the one time you are temporarily not available, will be the occasion when a serious patient related event will need your urgent input.

Box 2.3: *European working time directive (EWTD)*

- In 1998, the UK government agreed to implement the EWTD as health and safety legislation
- Since August 2004, no doctor should be working more than 58 hours a week
- By August 2007, this has to be reduced to 56 hours and to 49 hours by August 2009
- Many doctors will be forced to work full shifts
- Increasing use of non-medical staff to free up doctor's time

Box 2.4: *Key elements to minimize medical workload at night*

- Work within a multi-disciplinary, competency based team
- Upskill ward staff to minimize reliance on the night team
- Reduce duplication
- Take away inappropriate tasks
- Effective bleep or call policies
- Better use of new technologies, e.g. digital imaging

WARD REFERRALS (Box 2.6)

'I don't know anything about dermatology.' For some reason hospital doctors feel able to boast about their lack of knowledge of dermatology in a way that would be unthinkable if they were talking about other specialties. As a consequence of the minimal exposure to the specialty during undergraduate and postgraduate training, you will find that ward referrals form a large part of the daily workload. The JCHMT recommend that the trainee must have a regular commitment to seeing hospital inpatient referrals during their four years of higher medical training.

Although the temptation is to defer, the general consensus is that you should try and review ward patients on the day of referral. Procrastinating runs the risk of accumulating increasing numbers of referrals which would need to be accommodated outside normal hours and therefore influencing the management of these patients.

Liaising with the dermatology consultant on call is helpful for both patient welfare and specialist registrar education. With time, it is likely that you will be given increasing responsibility for carrying out consultations independently, although consultant advice should always be readily available.

INPATIENT CARE

Not all dermatology departments will have a dedicated ward with protected beds for their patients. Commonly, a lot of skin units will compete with acute medicine for available bed occupancy. Inpatient care is undoubtedly more focused and productive when performed by trained dermatology nurses who have the experience, expertise and time to treat and educate patients.

Box 2.5: On-call cover — best practice

- Have a well organized diary system for recording on-call commitments
- Ensure switchboard is aware of any changes
- Ensure that both parties fully understand the swap
- Record all swaps in writing
- The department should have accurate contact details readily available

---

Box 2.6: Ward referrals

- Try to attend to these on the day of referral
- ICU and paediatrics will expect prompt assessment
- Biopsies are best performed during normal working hours
- Write a concise and informed management plan in the notes
- If unsure, seek consultant advice
- Patients may need reviewing after initial assessment

It is likely that the dermatology ward will be medically staffed by a senior house officer (SHO) who will be responsible for the day-to-day running of the ward. The specialist registrar will supervise the SHO, be directly involved in patient management decisions, and will lead their own ward rounds. It is the SpR's role to support the consultant on their ward round. It is essential to ensure all decisions from previous consultant ward rounds have been actioned and all available investigations are to hand.

DAYCASE TREATMENT

An intermediate form of treatment, between outpatient and inpatient care, is daycase treatment. As the name implies, this part of the overall care plan is designed to offer specialist treatment without the need to admit the patient. The unit is typically staffed by senior experienced nurses who are able to provide one-to-one care and give informed advice and educational support to patients. There are advantages to using this service (Box 2.7).

It is important to identify in clinics which patients would be suitable for daycare and to liaise with senior staff running the unit to ensure full co-operation. It is essential that expectations from the treatment are realistic and are explained to the patient at the point of referral.

PRIMARY HEALTHCARE

General practitioners are aware of the huge prevalence of skin disease, which can account for up to 20% of all consultations, and this heavy workload is compounded by the deficiencies in their dermatological training.

It is useful for trainees to develop an understanding of the organization, problems and expectations present in primary healthcare. Specialist registrars will vary in their exposure to general practice prior to higher professional training. The majority of undergraduate courses now contain considerable general practice experience. The JCHMT recommends that those trainees with minimal exposure to primary healthcare should spend a *few* sessions in general practice in order to familiarize themselves with the work.

Apart from appreciating the presentation and management of dermatological problems in the primary care setting and understanding more about the organization of a health centre and its referral process, as a specialist trainee you would be able to provide teaching

---

Box 2.7: *Advantages of daycase treatment*

- Can avoid unnecessary admissions to hospital
- Allows for controlled, supervised application of treatment
- Reinforces learning points for patients and carers
- Allows for initial regular review without the need for outpatient appointments

sessions for the practice which may incorporate demonstrations of minor surgery or discussions surrounding the management of more complex cases.

MANAGEMENT SKILLS

Newly appointed consultants often describe the transition from trainee to consultant as 'dramatic'. As a group, they commonly state that they have been poorly prepared for seniority, in particular with regards to management issues. New consultants find that they need to know a great deal about the structure and history of the NHS, the trust and the department in which they work than when they were specialist registrars.

Although the JCHMT stipulates that the trainee should acquire the skills and knowledge necessary to understand the administrative structure and function of the NHS and to be able to familiarize business plans accordingly, in the majority of cases, little exposure is possible.

There are management courses available to the trainee that are often mandatory for completion of training; however, this limited preparation is insufficient. There may be moves to smooth the transition from trainee to consultant by incorporating programmed increase in managerial responsibilities for senior specialist registrars.

Management skills that are useful to acquire include time management, handling complaints, clinical risk management, clinical governance, personal development plans and appraisal.

TIME MANAGEMENT

For the majority of us, Parkinson's Law rules — work expands to fill the time available.

Differentiating between what is urgent and what is important

Successful time management starts with being aware of the difference between things that are urgent and those that are important, both at work and out of work. Urgent situations require speedy action and make pressing demands on time, but they are not necessarily important. For example, a patient comes into your dermatology outpatient clinic screaming and shouting. This is an urgent situation that requires immediate action. However, tasks or activities that can be defined as important matter greatly and may not require instant action but will have considerable effects. For example, professional exams are important because of the consequences and impact on a trainee's career and earning potential.

Meetings

Meetings are a common time-wasting activity in many organizations. Surveys show that the average manager spends:

- About 17 hours a week in meetings.
- Six hours in planning time.
- 'Incalculable' hours on follow-up work.

In some cases meetings are held simply because managers feel 'it's good to talk'. This may be so, but it can also be expensive, especially when other people monopolize meetings and work to their own private agendas. If you cannot justify your attendance at a meeting, then do not attend or consider alternative ways of gaining access to the information that will be presented.

Interruptions

Other people will make unnecessary demands on your time. You can protect yourself from unwanted or lengthy interruptions, or both, by:

- Keeping your office door closed.
- Standing when people enter your office to signal that you are busy.
- Removing seats from your office or keeping them 'occupied' with objects.
- Making people aware of your time limits.

Delegation

Many people fail to delegate because of the mistaken belief that the best way to make sure a job is done is to do it themselves. Good delegation helps other trainees to learn and develop new skills and also frees up your time to enable you to perform important tasks. Delegation is not to be confused with dumping. Successful delegation is based on a planned strategy, rather than offloading work at the last minute.

COMPLAINTS

Complaints can be distressing and upsetting experiences. Patients are no longer passive consumers of the care provided by their doctors. Improved education, increased expectations, the internet, and blanket media coverage of rare and extreme cases may explain the increasing number of complaints.

Most doctors will face at least one complaint during their professional lifetimes and many will come across several. Numerous complaints arise from simple confusion. However, misunderstandings with poor communication feature in most complaints referred to the medical defence societies (Box 2.8).

Once you have received a complaint it is vital to get the basic approach to handling this situation correct:

- Do not take criticisms personally.
- Act quickly and efficiently.
- Be willing to listen and sympathize.

- Provide an apology where appropriate.
- Give assurance that steps have been taken to prevent a recurrence.

If you are unsure of how to proceed when a complaint arises, get in touch with your medical defence organization. It can advise you of all the stages of the complaints procedure, including the local resolution process, and can help with your response. Remember never alter medical records at a later date. This is even more important if there has been a complaint.

In summary, whenever approached regarding a complaint, always give a full, factual and clinical account of your management of the patient, based on the records and your memory of the events. It is important to remember that apologizing for what happened is not an admission of guilt or liability.

CLINICAL GOVERNANCE AND CLINICAL RISK MANAGEMENT

Clinical governance is defined by the Department of Health (DoH) as:

> A framework through which NHS organizations are accountable for continuously improving the quality of their services and safeguarding high standards of care, by creating an environment in which excellence in clinical care will flourish.

Thus, clinical governance aims to ensure that patients get effective and safe treatment and that the risks associated with clinical care are prevented or minimized. The improvement of quality of services can be undertaken through various activities (Box 2.9).

Healthcare risk is the probability of a patient suffering harm from a clinical activity. The risk may be clinical (wrong diagnosis, wrong treatment, faulty equipment), environmental

---

Box 2.8: Minimizing communication misunderstandings

- Set out what you intend to do in clear and simple language
- Avoid medical jargon when communicating with patients
- Make sure patients understand — ask them to repeat what you have told them
- Obtain informed consent
- Write clearly in medical notes
- Provide information leaflets where appropriate

Box 2.9: Quality improvement activities

- Clinical guidelines/evidence-based practice
- Continuing professional development/life-long learning
- Clinical audit
- Effective monitoring of clinical care
- Research and development

(slippery floors, falling objects), or organizational (poor supplies, inadequate staff). Risks are minimized by recognition and prevention.

PERSONAL DEVELOPMENT PLANS

The Department of Health (DoH) paper in 1998 on continuing professional development (CPD) suggested a move from unstructured, traditional continuing medical education (CME) to the accreditation of structured personal development plans (PDPs).

A PDP is a tool to encourage life-long learning and identify any areas for further development. Reflecting on your specific learning needs forms the basis of a PDP by identifying educational and training needs.

The PDP is encountered by trainees when they meet up with their educational supervisors. It is recommended that trainee and trainer should meet at least three times a year. The initial session is to outline a PDP for the forthcoming year; importantly, identifying learning needs. The subsequent encounters are to assess how successful this training plan has been.

Box 2.10 outlines how these learning needs may have arisen. PDPs are learning contracts with agreed educational targets, which can then be used in the revalidation process. The evidence of this continuing learning forms the framework of the JCHMT logbook which trainees must keep up to date.

APPRAISAL

This is an essential component of a specialist registrar's training programme. These opportunities, when trainer and trainee are in discussion, allow trainers to make comments upon their perception of the trainee's performance and whether the set objectives in the PDP have been achieved.

Trainers should provide careful and constructive feedback, backed up with specific examples. This will reinforce the concept of appraisal as a positive experience.

Trainees should be encouraged to give their perceptions of the training they have received without fear of reprisal. They should suggest realistic ways in which difficult areas of their training could be improved.

Box 2.10

Learning needs may have arisen from:

- Awkward moments with colleagues
- Important events, e.g. British Association of Dermatologists Annual meetings
- External priorities, e.g. clinical governance
- Educational appraisal with tutor

At the end of the appraisal interview, the registrar should leave with objectives having been set for their next posts and a record of these should form part of their educational supervisor meeting reports within their logbooks (Box 2.11).

PERFORMANCE ASSESSMENT

Assessment of the performance of doctors has become an important issue as a result of high profile cases and the redesign of medical training.

The Royal Colleges of Physicians (UK) have developed three methods of performance assessment.

a) Mini-CEX (clinical evaluation exercise),
b) DOPS (Directly Observed Procedural Skills),
c) MSF (Multi-sourced Feedback or 360 degree assessment).

Mini-CEX (clinical evaluation exercise)

The skills which are being assessed during the mini-CEX include:

- Medical interviewing skills
- Physical examination skills
- Consideration for patient/professionalism
- Clinical judgement
- Counselling and communication skills
- Organization/efficiency
- Overall clinical competence.

Each domain is scored from 1–9 where 1–3 = unsatisfactory, 4–6 = satisfactory, and 7–9 = above average. Mini-CEXs can be carried out both in outpatient and inpatient settings. It is recommended that SpRs should be assessed by several consultants during their course of training. The suggestion by the JCHMT is that each mini-CEX should take approximately 15 minutes and the trainees should have a minimum of four mini-CEXs per year.

Box 2.11: Appraisal points

- Appraisal is an integral part of training
- It should be used constructively by both trainee and trainer
- Setting objectives early is a key to success
- Trainees must be able to discuss their development
- Appraisal requires time and should be undertaken in protected time, set aside and identified in advance to the trainee
- Use of personal development plans should be encouraged
- Appraisal is confidential between trainee and trainer

DOPS (Directly Observed Procedural Skills)

This focuses on the core skills that SpRs require when undertaking a clinical practical procedure. A particular procedure is decided upon by the trainee and consultant. The consultant then directly observes the trainee performing the task in a normal environment and the SpR is then scored as outlined above.

MSF (Multi-sourced Feedback or 360 degree assessment)

This is a method of assessing generic skills such as communication, leadership, team working, teaching, punctuality and reliability. This then allows objective systematic collection and feedback of performance data on the trainee, which is derived from a number of stakeholders in their performance, i.e. nurses, other doctors, secretaries, other clerical staff and other allied health professionals. On average, the data from 20 forms are put together to provide the SpR with structured feedback about their performance.

TEACHING

As a specialist registrar, you will be expected to undertake teaching duties. Your heart should not necessarily sink at this prospect! This process can often be very rewarding. Medical students are attached to dermatology for a short period of time, usually one or two weeks. With this brief exposure to the subject it is imperative that learning experiences are maximized.

Teaching in dermatology can take the form of bedside learning, slide tutorials, case histories, outpatient instruction and possibly e-learning using online techniques, for example, registrars may facilitate tutorials to students via academic dermatology websites.

What makes a good teacher?

The focus of instruction should always be on student learning, not faculty teaching. Too often clinicians concentrate on what they want students to know rather than what they actually need to know as practising doctors.

Good teachers do not talk as much as their less effective colleagues do! This is because good teachers involve the learners — asking questions, framing cases to solve, forming small groups for discussion, asking for the views of the learners, pausing to allow students to think. When they do talk, good teachers use words efficiently. They make concepts and principles simple and clear.

While it is necessary for a teacher to be highly knowledgeable in their field, I believe it is perhaps more important to show enthusiasm and interest in teaching that subject. This excitement for learning is demonstrated by being a well organized and expressive lecturer who presents information concisely and involves students in problem solving. As a teacher you want to create an environment where curiosity is encouraged, problems related to the discipline are solved and feedback is solicited from the learners.

In summary:

- Be enthusiastic about your teaching.
- Prepare well for your teaching.
- Teach knowledge in the context of solving authentic medical problems.
- Use and solicit feedback.

Further reading

Department of Health. NHS Complaints reform: making things right. London: DoH, 2003.

Evans A, Ali S, Singleton C, et al. The effectiveness of personal education plans in continuing professional development: an evaluation. Med Teach 2002; 24:79–84.

Hooke R. Junior doctors should be given more opportunities to participate in management. BMJ 2002; 325 (suppl):S63.

Markert RJ. What makes a good teacher? Lessons from teaching medical students. Academic Medicine 2001; 761:809–810.

McGuire R. Successful time management. BMJ 2003; 326 (suppl):S117.

Mowat D. Management training for the aspiring consultant. BMJ 2002; 325 (suppl):S61.

O'Hara J, Carter Y. PDPs – helpful tool or junk? Update 2002; 64:342–344.

Useful websites

www.jchmt.org.uk/assessment

www.bad.org.uk/healthcare/competency_assessments

An introduction to dermatopathology

3

Richard A. Logan

INTRODUCTION

A sound working knowledge of dermatopathology is fundamentally important to the practising dermatologist. It assists the development of a logical approach to clinical diagnosis. It helps to decide when, where and how to take a skin biopsy. Furthermore it allows a more productive working relationship between dermatologist and histopathologist.

Whether consciously or not, dermatologists choose their specialty because they have an aptitude for visual pattern recognition. Histopathologists have this too, so it is not a surprise that significant numbers of dermatologists are interested and skilled in dermatopathology.

Crowded undergraduate curricula seem to provide little opportunity for the systematic study of histopathology. This chapter therefore concentrates on basic concepts in dermatopathology. These concepts are expanded in a recent, more detailed discussion.[1]

THE MAGNIFICATION HIERARCHY

Diagnosis may be achieved by examining the skin at increasing degrees of magnification:

- *Naked eye* — most clinical diagnoses are made without further investigation.

- *Dermatoscopy* — recent introduction of hand-held devices allows instant magnification up to ×10. This is useful in assessing pigmented lesions but requires practice to learn a complete new range of pattern recognition. Its principal advantage is to increase diagnostic confidence concerning the need for surgical excision.

- *Light microscopy* — this remains the 'gold standard' in the diagnostic process allowing the skin to be magnified up to ×1000.

- *Electron microscopy* — this is now less often used in diagnostic dermatopathology because newer and simpler immunohistochemical techniques are often able to provide sufficient information, e.g. in the field of epidermolysis bullosa diagnosis.

Although skin histopathology is the technique most relied upon for accurate diagnosis, not infrequently a pathology report is received along these lines:

> Skin showing a moderate degree of irregular epidermal acanthosis with patchy parakeratosis. There is a mild perivascular lymphocytic infiltrate but no true vasculitis. The changes are mild and non-specific.

Thus histopathology does not always provide a specific diagnosis. Clinical judgement remains paramount. However, even when a report is not diagnostic, it often helps to eliminate some diagnoses.

HELP YOUR PATHOLOGIST

It is said of computers 'rubbish in, rubbish out'. In much the same way, to get the most helpful report from our pathologists it is essential to assist them in a number of important ways, by:

- Choosing the most appropriate lesion to biopsy.
- Using the correct biopsy technique.
- Collecting and labelling the specimen.
- Providing enough information on the pathology request form.
- Discussing difficult cases.

The most appropriate lesion to biopsy

- As a general rule, the newer the lesion the more appropriate it is for biopsy. Older lesions are more likely to have been modified, for example by scratching or secondary bacterial infection. This is particularly true for inflammatory bullous diseases such as bullous pemphigoid.
- For eruptions on the legs such as suspected vasculitis, biopsy the highest lesion, because gravitational effects on the cutaneous vasculature are more marked lower on the leg and these can cause diagnostic confusion.
- Do not biopsy the middle of a scarring condition such as morphoea or cicatricial alopecia. Take an ellipse of skin from the actively inflamed edge of the lesion to include normal skin for comparison.

The correct biopsy technique (p. 220)

- Punch biopsy — this delivers a small cylinder of skin, usually 3–4 mm in diameter. Its main uses are:
  - to establish a diagnosis from a tumour, e.g. basal cell carcinoma, where further definitive treatment will follow;
  - for investigating inflammatory diseases where there is unlikely to be major variation in pathological changes in different parts of the lesion, e.g. discoid lupus erythematosus, vasculitis, Jessner's lymphocytic infiltrate;
  - to remove very small lesions;

- to produce minimal scarring in cosmetically important areas such as the face;
- for obtaining specimens for immunofluorescence (see later).
- Punch biopsy has *important disadvantages* relevant to pathological assessment:
  - the specimen is small which may lead to it not being sectioned perpendicular to the epidermis;
  - small size can lead to sampling error in lesions where there is a gradation of pathological changes in different parts of the lesion, e.g. bullous conditions; suspected lentigo maligna; the edge of ulcers;
  - in conditions where the pathology is suspected to be deep in the skin, e.g. panniculitis, the punch may not remove sufficient deep material.
- Curettage — this is widely used for removing superficial lesions such as seborrhoeic and viral warts, solar keratoses and also for debulking tumours prior to excision of the base. Because the curettage specimen is fragmented and variably orientated, the pathologist can only comment on the likely nature of the pathology but is unable to offer an opinion on the adequacy of tumour removal. It is common, for example, for reports on curetted Bowen's disease to include a caveat regarding the possibility of foci of invasive squamous carcinoma. Keratoacanthoma (KA) is a special case in point. If the lesion is fragmented during the process of curettage, the overall architectural arrangement of the tumour is lost (Figure 3.1). This makes it even more difficult for the pathologist to differentiate between KA and squamous carcinoma.
- Shave excision — with this technique superficial skin is removed using either a scalpel blade or razor blade cutting horizontally, parallel to the skin surface. Its main application is in the removal of cellular naevi, when almost always the lower intradermal parts of the naevus are left behind. This does not usually matter clinically, unless the naevus was pigmented. In this case the wound may heal with an unusual pattern of repigmentation. This can cause clinical concern about the possibility of malignant melanoma, and if the area is subsequently re-excised it may show atypical melanocytic changes (pseudo-melanoma).
- 'Ellipse' biopsy — this is the standard and most widely used technique. It is appropriate for the removal of tumours in that it allows the pathologist to examine the periphery of the excised specimen and thus comment on the likelihood of the adequacy of removal. It should be employed if the pathology is likely to be deeper in the skin. It should also be used for diagnostic biopsies where there is likely to be a gradation of pathology from the

Figure 3.1
Architecture of keratoacanthoma. The lesion shows symmetry which is only apparent to the pathologist if it is removed intact.

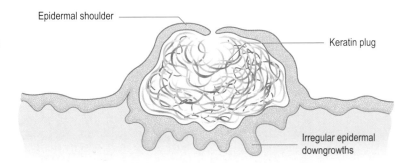

Epidermal shoulder

Keratin plug

Irregular epidermal downgrowths

normal skin into the centre of the lesion, e.g. ulcers, scarring and blistering disorders. In this case the long axis of the biopsy should be at right angles to the margin of the lesion to include normal skin (Figure 3.2).

Collecting and labelling the specimen

Regardless of the type of biopsy it is important to minimize trauma to the excised skin. The local anaesthetic should be injected into the fat under the skin to be removed, to avoid haemorrhagic changes and other distortions in the dermis from the passage of the injecting needle. If urticaria pigmentosa is suspected, the local anaesthetic should be injected around rather than under the lesion to reduce the risk of degranulating the mast cells. Crush artefact (Figure 3.3) is very common and is due to the skin being gripped by dissecting forceps. This can be avoided by holding the skin at one end (preferably the normal skin) or better by the use of a skin hook.

In some situations it is wise to take more than one biopsy, especially if lesions have different morphology at separate sites. This is especially true if cutaneous T-cell lymphoma is suspected. In this condition, even when there is strong clinical suspicion of the diagnosis, it can take many biopsies, sometimes over years, before the diagnosis is confirmed histologically.

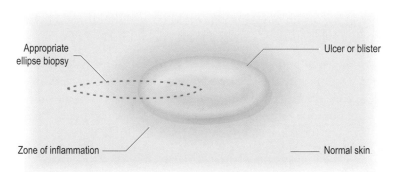

Figure 3.2
The correct way to biopsy a blister or an ulcer.

Appropriate ellipse biopsy

Ulcer or blister

Zone of inflammation

Normal skin

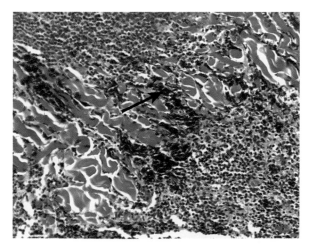

Figure 3.3
Crush artefact. Biopsy of follicular lymphoma. Arrow indicates an area where lymphocytes have been crushed during biopsy.

For routine histopathology the excised skin specimen is placed into a specimen pot containing 10% neutral buffered formalin. Specimens for immunofluorescence should be placed in Michel's transport medium (Table 3.1) which preserves antigens and antibodies in the specimen for up to 6 months.[2] This avoids the need for such specimens to be snap-frozen and transported in liquid nitrogen.

Occasionally it is also necessary to send parts of a biopsy for additional tests such as bacteriological or fungal culture. It is tempting to remove a skin 'ellipse' and then divide this up into smaller pieces. This should be avoided as it traumatizes the main specimen making histological assessment more difficult. It is preferable to take two samples and divide the second into halves for further tests.

It is vitally important that the details of the patient tally on the histology request form and the specimen pot. If more than one specimen has been removed then they should be put into separate pots and the forms and pots labelled with an identifying letter and the site of the biopsy. This is to avoid confusion at a later date when one biopsy may turn out to be malignant and the other benign.

WHAT HAPPENS TO MY BIOPSY IN THE LABORATORY?

It is important to know how a skin biopsy is processed in the laboratory. This aids the understanding of some of the limitations, artefacts and delays inherent in the system.

For routine histopathology skin biopsies are initially placed into formalin fixative. From receipt in the laboratory to the specimen being ready for histopathological assessment takes on average about 48 hours, although occasionally it is possible to have a result in 24 hours. Frozen sections are rarely used in dermatology apart from the assessment of micrographic (Mohs) sections (p. 240) but these specimens can be assessed in 20 minutes.

Depending on the size of the biopsy and when it is received in the laboratory, the specimen will remain in formalin for between 3 and 18 hours (longer at weekends). The formalin makes the specimen firm to facilitate cutting up into a size small enough to allow the process of paraffin wax embedding.

For curettings, the pieces are processed 'all in'. It follows that they will be orientated in many different directions. This means later that the pathologist will not be able to make any statement on the adequacy of excision of, for example, a curetted basal cell carcinoma. A

Table 3.1: Michel's fixative for immunofluorescence	
Ammonium sulphate	55 g in 100 mL buffer
Buffer	Distilled water, 87.5 mL 1 mol/L potassium citrate (pH 7), 2.5 mL 0.1 mol/L magnesium sulphate, 5 mL 0.1 mol/L ethyl maleimide, 5 mL Mix 1:2 with 1 mol/L potassium hydroxide to pH 7

small punch biopsy or shave biopsy will also be processed 'all in'. However, here it is usual for the technician to be able to orientate the specimen so that the epidermis and dermis are correctly positioned for later sectioning. 'Ellipse' biopsies are usually sectioned longitudinally before processing. However, for larger specimens (e.g. removal of malignant melanoma) the biopsy is divided as shown in Figure 3.4. A narrow transverse section will be taken from the middle of the biopsy, with possibly up to six or nine further transverse sections (levels) for more detailed analysis (e.g. Breslow tumour thickness assessment). The remnants of the original four quarters of the biopsy are sectioned longitudinally.[3] Examination of several levels may lead to a delay in receipt of the report on a suspicious pigmented lesion.

Malorientation of the specimen at the 'cut-up' stage will lead later to the sample being sectioned at an angle not perpendicular to the skin surface. This can make the epidermis look thicker than it actually was (Figure 3.5) and also leads to inaccurate assessments of tumour thickness. The process of fixing and subsequent dehydration causes shrinkage artefact. Thus histological assessments of the measurement of excision margins are not exactly the same as the true surgical margins, which should be measured at the time of biopsy.

After 'cut-up' the pieces of the biopsy are then placed in 3 mm thick cassettes to allow the process of wax embedding. This takes up to 16 hours and involves progressive dehydration of the specimen through several alcohol baths, 'clearing' in xylene (to remove the alcohol) and then embedding in paraffin wax to form a block. Sections of 4 µ thickness are then cut from the block with a microtome and floated onto a warm water bath from which they are picked up onto glass slides for staining.

Staining techniques

The standard technique for routine histology is haematoxylin and eosin staining (H & E). This process is automated and takes about 20 minutes. Nuclei stain blue-purple, connective tissue and red blood cells (RBCs) pink-red. This stain is sufficient for most diagnostic purposes but does have some limitations. It cannot differentiate between different pigments, and does not show some structures such as elastic fibres and micro-organisms such as bacteria which require additional staining techniques.

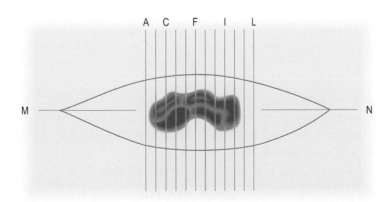

Figure 3.4
Method of taking step sections ('levels') through a biopsy of a suspicious pigmented lesion.

Figure 3.5
Tangential sectioning. This can give an erroneous net-like appearance and an incorrect impression of epidermal thickness.

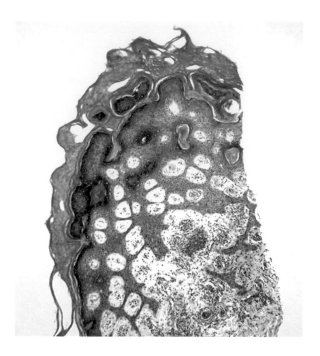

Some suspected diagnoses prompt additional stains to be carried out immediately, e.g. periodic acid-Schiff (PAS) for fungi. More often, additional stains may be carried out after the slides have been examined by the pathologist, e.g. Ziehl–Neelsen for acid fast bacilli, if the pathology is granulomatous. Some of the stains used more commonly for dermatopathology[4] are shown in Table 3.2.

Examining the slide

There are several steps in the microscopic assessment of a histology slide and each practitioner will develop their own method. Briefly these steps are:

- Naked eye:
  - Check that the label on the slide matches the details on the request form.
  - Hold the slide up to the light: how many sections are there, how big are they, are they from the same specimen?
  - Is there more than one specimen from the patient, and if so, which one are you looking at?
  - What is the dominant staining colour?
- Low power (scanning magnification: ×2.5–4 objective lens):
  - Is there any obvious pathology?
  - Where is the pathology: is it in the epidermis, the dermis or both; is it in the fat?
  - What is the pattern of the pathology?[5]
  - Look at all the sections on the slide: do they differ significantly?
- Higher power (×10–100 objective):
  - Study the cellular detail.

Table 3.2: Some of the histochemical stains commonly used in dermatopathology

Stain	Tissue	Colour reaction
Periodic acid-Schiff (PAS)	Glycogen (e.g. Degos' acanthoma)	Magenta
	Mucopolysaccharide (e.g. basement membrane; fungal walls)	
Grocott	Fungal wall	Black
Methenamine silver	Gram +ve bacteria	Blue/violet
	Gram −ve	Red/pink
Ziehl–Neelsen	Acid fast bacilli	Red
Wade–Fite	Leprosy bacilli	
Alcian blue	Acid mucopolysaccharides, e.g. mucinoses; extra-mammary Paget's	Blue
Toluidine blue	Acid mucopolysaccharides, e.g. mast cell granules	Purple 'metachromasia'
Giemsa	Mast cells	Purple 'metachromasia'
	Leishmania	Blue
Van Gieson	Collagen	Red
	Muscle/nerve	Yellow
Acid orcein-Giemsa	Collagen	Pink
	Elastic fibres	Brown/black
	Mast cell granules	Purple
	Melanin	Black
Perl's (Prussian blue)	Iron (usually in haemosiderin)	Blue
Congo red	Amyloid (best to confirm using additional technique such as thioflavin T or occasionally electron microscopy)	Red (with green birefringence under polarized light)
Gomori's silver	Reticulin (especially for assessing growth pattern in melanocytic lesions)	Black
Chloroacetate esterase	Mast cells	Red

– Are the cells homogeneous or a mixed population?

– Is the process inflammatory, neoplastic or otherwise?

– If neoplastic, is it benign or malignant?

– Are further techniques (e.g. immunocytochemistry/immunofluorescence) needed to clarify either the type of cells or the immunopathology?

• Return to low power — have you missed anything?

REGIONAL VARIATIONS OF NORMAL SKIN STRUCTURE

Normal skin has significant variations according to body site which can be summarized as follows:

- Scalp — this has large hair follicles with sebaceous glands. The hair bulbs are often in the subcutaneous fat (Figure 3.6)
- Face — this shows smaller hair follicles and prominent sebaceous glands. The epidermis is thinner than on the scalp with a less well developed rete ridge pattern. Striated muscle fibres may be seen in the upper dermis in biopsies taken from around the mouth and eye.
- Axilla — hair follicles and apocrine glands are evident and the epidermis may be folded (papillomatosis).
- Trunk — the dermis is much thicker than other parts of the body, especially on the back.
- Mucous membranes — the cells of the Malpighian layer of the epidermis are large and pale. There is very little stratum corneum which usually retains its nuclei (physiological parakeratosis).
- Scrotum and nipple — here the epidermis is papillomatous and smooth muscle fibres can be seen in the superficial dermis.
- Lower leg — in older patients, especially in the presence of venous hypertension, the dermal capillary network becomes dilated and tortuous. This can lead to a histological appearance of increased numbers of small capillaries in the papillary dermis.
- Palms and soles — the epidermis is thick with a well-marked rete ridge pattern. The stratum corneum is considerably thickened (Figure 3.7).

COMMON DERMATOPATHOLOGY TERMS

There is a large vocabulary used in the description of skin histopathology. It is perhaps easiest to consider these terms 'from the outside inwards'.

Figure 3.6
Scalp biopsy showing terminal hair follicles.

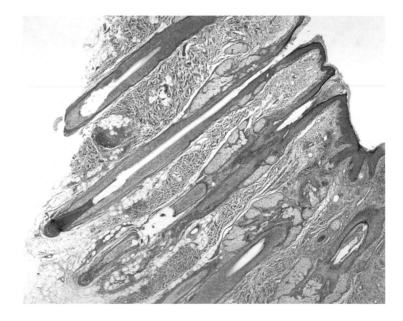

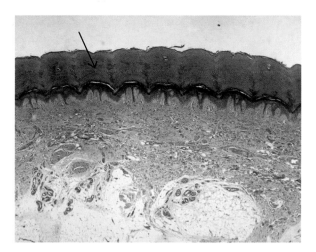

Figure 3.7
Biopsy of palmar/sole skin. Note the thick stratum corneum (black arrow).

Epidermis

Acanthosis is thickening of the epidermis. It may be even and regular as in psoriasis, or uneven as in chronic eczema or prurigo nodularis. Thinning of the epidermis is *atrophy*, seen for example in lichen sclerosus or after topical steroid therapy. When the epidermis is thrown into folds it is known as *papillomatosis*. This can be physiological as in the axilla or pathological, e.g. viral wart.

Stratum corneum: the normal pattern is 'basket weave' *orthokeratosis*, where the nuclei have been shed from the corneocytes. *Hyperkeratosis* describes any condition where the stratum corneum is thickened. In *parakeratosis*, nuclei are retained in the corneocytes. A large range of disturbances can produce parakeratosis, especially inflammatory diseases such as eczema and psoriasis. It is physiological on mucous membranes. The collection together of serous exudates, bacteria and inflammatory cell debris on the surface is *crust*.

Stratum granulosum: hypergranulosis is thickening of this layer. It is typical of, but not exclusive to, lichen planus. *Epidermolytic hyperkeratosis* is a striking appearance where the granular layer is thickened and shows increased coarse granulation and perinuclear vacuolation.

Stratum spinosum: widening of the gap between keratinocytes with oedema fluid is *spongiosis*, typically seen in acute forms of eczema. Coalescence of this fluid may lead to vesicles or even *bullae*. When the cells lose their inter-cellular adhesion and fall apart from each other it is known as *acantholysis*, a change typical of pemphigus, Darier's disease and Hailey–Hailey disease. *Dyskeratosis* is an abnormal pattern of premature keratinization of keratinocytes. The cytoplasm is pinker than normal and nuclei usually small and dark (*pyknosis*). It is typical of squamous carcinoma, Bowen's and Darier's diseases. *Exocytosis* is the term used when inflammatory or other cells permeate from the dermis into the epidermis, e.g. lymphocytes in eczema and psoriasis. Atypical lymphocytes may collect in the epidermis in cutaneous T-cell lymphoma by a process known as *epidermotropism*, where they may coalesce to form small *Pautrier microabscesses*. *Necrolysis* is death of all or part of the epidermis as in erythema multiforme or toxic epidermal necrolysis.

Basal layer: this is damaged in conditions such as lichen planus and lupus erythematosus. The cells may initially show *vacuolar degeneration* and later die to form *colloid (Civatte) bodies* which are rounded and eosinophilic. The shape of the rete ridges may be altered to a *'saw-tooth' pattern* in lichen planus. Increased numbers of melanocytes are seen in *lentigo*. A *villus (pl. villi)* is an upwards projection of dermal papilla retaining a single layer of basal cells. It may be seen in various blistering disorders such as pemphigus.

Dermis

Papillary: this is often the site of inflammatory changes. An intense band-like concentration of lymphocytes in this area and the adjacent upper dermis is called *lichenoid infiltration*. It is seen in lichen planus, other lichenoid conditions and cutaneous T-cell lymphoma. Collections here of polymorphonuclear cells with oedema are called *papillary tip microabscesses* and are typical of dermatitis herpetiformis. The absence of inflammation in this area with abnormalities deeper in the dermis is called a *Grenz zone*. Collections of melanocytic naevus cells in this area are called *theques*, and are seen in junctional and compound melanocytic naevi. *Pigmentary incontinence* is the presence in the upper dermis of melanin, either free or phagocytosed in melanophages. It usually signifies previous damage to the basal layer as in lichen planus.

Reticular: elastotic degeneration affects the papillary and upper reticular dermis due to damage from ultraviolet or less commonly ionizing radiation. *Fibrinoid change* is the deposition of eosinophilic material around dermal blood vessel walls most commonly due to necrotizing vasculitis. *Hyaline change* is amorphous pale pink material seen for example in the upper dermis in lichen sclerosus and around blood vessels in porphyria. *Nuclear dust (leukocytoclasis)* is fine stippled basophilic material near blood vessels, seen typically in hypersensitivity angiitis (leukocytoclastic vasculitis). *Storiform (curlicue) patterning* is the description of the way cells in dermatofibroma and dermatofibrosarcoma protruberans twist amongst collagen fibres to resemble a rush-mat. *Desmoplasia* is sclerosis of dermal connective tissue in reaction to tumours such as morphoeic basal cell carcinoma or desmoplastic malignant melanoma. *Necrobiosis* arises from granulomatous disorders leading to the death of dermal connective tissue. There is a zone of pale homogenized tissue usually surrounded by a 'palisade' of mixed histiocytic cells. This change may be seen in granuloma annulare, necrobiosis lipoidica and rheumatoid nodule.

Subcutis (fat)

Panniculitis is the term used to describe inflammation of the fat, which can either be in the fat lobules (*lobular panniculitis*) or in the intervening fibrous septae (*septal panniculitis*). In practice both patterns are often seen together. Panniculitis has a wide range of causes, the most common being erythema nodosum.

HIGH POWER CYTOLOGY

After studying the slide at low and high power and observing the overall pattern of pathology, it is usually necessary to look carefully at the appearance of the individual cells. Of course the most important decision to be made is whether the condition is benign or malignant.

Inflammatory conditions may contain a variety of different cell types (pleomorphism) such as lymphocytes, histiocytes, plasma cells and eosinophils. Alternatively the infiltrate may be monomorphic and consist of almost pure populations of one cell type, e.g. lymphocytes or neutrophils. Some of the important features of these commoner cells are shown in Table 3.3.

Table 3.3: Common cell types in inflammatory conditions

Cell type	Size	Cytology	Examples	Comments
Lymphocyte	7–12 μ	Small, round, darkly staining nucleus with thin rim of cytoplasm	The predominant cell in many inflammatory skin diseases; lymphomas and leukaemias	T and B lymphocytes indistinguishable on light microscopy but distinguished by immunohistochemical techniques
Neutrophil	10–15 μ	Multilobed nucleus; more cytoplasm than lymphocyte containing lysosomal granules; cytoplasm appears pink	Pus-forming infections, e.g. *Staph* abscesses; sterile pyodermas, e.g. pyoderma gangrenosum; leukocytoclastic vasculitis	Phagocytic cells — cytoplasmic granules not visible on light microscopy
Eosinophil	12–17 μ	Nucleus has only two lobes; cytoplasm is eosinophilic and appears orange	'Drugs and bugs', i.e. insect bites, infestations and drug reactions; pemphigoid and pemphigus	Phagocytic cells — often seen in allergic reactions
Plasma cell	10 μ	Eccentric nucleus with 'clock face' pattern of chromatin; perinuclear pale halo in cytoplasm	Inflammatory conditions of hair-bearing skin and mucous membranes; late stage of granulomata; syphilis	Plasma cell is a specialized B lymphocyte dedicated to immunoglobulin production
'Histiocytes' (Tissue macrophages)	15–25 μ	Very variable. Fairly large cells, with a pale elongated nucleus. Cytoplasm pale. Shape varies from spindle-shaped to dendritic or epithelioid	Wide range of inflammatory, granulomatous, chronic infectious and neoplastic disorders, e.g. granuloma annulare; lupus vulgaris	Derived from circulating blood monocytes. Function is phagocytosis
Giant cells (GC) Three main types:	40–120 μ	1. Langhans' GC have horse-shoe arrangement of nuclei 2. Foreign body GC have random arrangement 3. Touton GC have central ring	Langhans': sarcoidosis and TB Foreign body: may contain ingested foreign material Touton: xanthomata and juvenile xanthogranuloma	

Features suggesting malignancy are:

- Variable size and shape of cells (pleomorphism).
- Variation in nuclear size and staining pattern; increase in nucleoli.
- Increased number of mitotic figures.
- Abnormal mitoses.
- Loss of polarity of epidermal cells — this is seen particularly in pre-malignant epidermal dysplasias such as solar keratoses and Bowen's disease as well as in frank malignancy such as squamous cell carcinoma.
- Invasion of neurovascular bundles.
- Single cell infiltration between collagen bundles.

FURTHER LABORATORY TESTS

Having examined the slide at low and high power the histological appearances may suggest the need for additional tests. These include:

- Examination of the slide under polarized light.
- Histochemical stains (Table 3.2).
- Immunopathological examination.[6]
  - Immunofluorescence.
  - Immunoenzyme methods.
- Molecular biological studies (cutaneous lymphoma).

Polarized light examination

Most light microscopes are equipped with a polarizing filter that can be turned to examine the specimen under polarized light. Refractile foreign material such as starch powder, suture material or urate crystals will shine brightly under these conditions. It is also used with Congo red staining to look for amyloid. Polarization should always be included in the assessment of a granulomatous tissue reaction.

Immunofluorescence (IF)

This is used to detect the presence and position of antigens in skin biopsies (direct IF). It can also be used to detect the presence of circulating antibody in serum (indirect IF). Its main application in dermatology is the evaluation of immunobullous diseases.

For direct IF a small skin biopsy (usually 3–4 mm punch) is best taken from skin which is not usually exposed to sunlight (e.g. inner arm). Alternatively it may be taken from non-lesional skin at least 2 cm away from the edge of a lesion. The specimen should preferably be placed in Michel's medium (Table 3.1) or snap-frozen in liquid nitrogen. It should *not* be placed in formalin which can degrade the antigens in question and make their retrieval more difficult.[7] After sectioning, the specimen is incubated with a rabbit derived anti-human antibody labelled with fluorochromes that fluoresce when examined under ultraviolet. Fluorescein is used to locate antigen and gives apple-green fluorescence, and rhodamine glows orange-red and is used as a 'counter stain' to show the position of epidermal nuclei. The patterns of fluorescence seen in various immunobullous diseases are shown in Table 3.4.

This technique can also be used as a prognostic indicator in the evaluation of cutaneous lupus erythematosus (lupus band test). The presence of one or more immunoreactants (other than IgM) on the basement membrane zone of non sun-exposed skin increases the likelihood of systemic involvement. The lupus band test has been less often used in recent years.

In indirect IF the patient's serum is incubated with an epidermal substrate (e.g. monkey oesophagus, human foreskin, rat bladder) to allow any antibody present to bind to epidermal substrate. Any bound human antibody is then detected by a second incubation with fluorochrome labelled anti-human antibody and examined as above. The main application of this technique is in the evaluation of bullous pemphigoid and pemphigus. The titre of antibody present correlates with disease activity in pemphigus but not in pemphigoid. To distinguish between bullous pemphigoid and its rarer, troublesome 'variant' epidermolysis bullosa acquisita, patients' serum can be incubated with salt-split skin as the substrate (Table 3.4).

In many smaller hospitals it is common practice for immunofluorescence studies to be carried out on 'batched' specimens. This is because reagents are expensive and the technique may only be carried out every 2–4 weeks. Thus the results of IF tests are often received later than the initial histopathology report.

Immunoenzyme methods[9]

The principle of this technique is similar to that of immunofluorescence. The difference is that instead of conjugating a diagnostic antibody to a fluorochrome it is conjugated to an

Table 3.4: Results of direct immunofluorescence

Disease	Immunoreactant(s)	Site	Pattern
Bullous pemphigoid	IgG and C3	Dermo-epidermal junction (DEJ) (epidermal side on salt-split skin)[8]	Linear
Epidermolysis bullosa acquisita	IgG and C3	DEJ (dermal side on salt-split skin)	Linear
Cicatricial pemphigoid	IgG and C3	DEJ	Linear
Herpes gestationis	C3	DEJ	Linear
Linear IgA disease	IgA	DEJ	Linear
Pemphigus	IgG and C3	Around epidermal cells	Net-like
Paraneoplastic pemphigus	{ IgG (occasionally C3) and/or IgG, C3 (occasionally IgM)	Around epidermal cells DEJ	Net-like and/or linear and granular
Dermatitis herpetiformis	IgA	Papillary tips	Granular and focal
Bullous lupus erythematosus	Many immunoglobulins, C3 and fibrin	DEJ	Linear homogeneous or non-homogeneous

enzyme, usually horseradish peroxidase (occasionally alkaline phosphatase). When the enzyme substrate is added, the substrate is broken down into coloured reaction product (brown for peroxidase, blue for alkaline phosphatase) at the site of binding of antibody on the section (Figure 3.8).

The advantage of this technique is that it can be used on paraffin-embedded sections and the reaction product does not decay with time. It is used to categorize the likely cell type on a section, and is particularly useful in diagnosing tumours. A large number of antibodies to different cell types have been developed in recent years, some of which are shown in Table 3.5.

Figure 3.8
Biopsy of malignant melanoma stained for S-100 (immunoperoxidase technique). Melanoma cells stain brown.

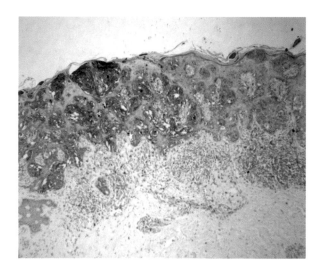

Table 3.5: A small selection of cell markers used in immunocytochemistry

Diagnostic group	Marker	Cell or tumour type
Poorly differentiated malignancy[10]	Cytokeratins (e.g. CAM 5.2; MNF 116) S-100; HMB-45; MART-1 LCA (leukocyte common antigen)	Carcinoma Melanoma Lymphoma
Lymphoma[11]	UCHL-1 L26 Ber-H2 (CD30)	Pan T-cell marker Pan B-cell marker Lymphomatoid papulosis and large cell lymphoma
Soft tissue neoplasms	S-100 Factor XIIIa Desmin Smooth muscle actin (SMA) CD-34	Neurofibroma; Schwannoma Dermal dendrocyte (dermatofibroma) Skeletal muscle Leiomyoma; glomus tumour Dermatofibrosarcoma protruberans
Small, blue cell tumours	LCA Cytokeratin S-100 Neurone specific enolase	Lymphoma Merkel cell tumour Melanoma Neuroblastoma
Vascular tumours	Factor VIII related antigen	Endothelium

Molecular biological studies[12]

These have a particular application in the investigation of cutaneous lymphomas.[13] Techniques such as Southern blot analysis and polymerase chain reaction (PCR) are employed to investigate the presence of specific clonal abnormalities of the T- and B-cell receptor genes. Both techniques involve the extraction of DNA from tissue samples, which can be either a skin biopsy or blood specimen. These tests are highly specialized and carried out in only a few reference laboratories. Results may take several weeks. Although the demonstration of the presence of a clonal T-cell receptor gene rearrangement can help in the diagnosis of cutaneous T-cell lymphoma, this cannot be regarded as the sole diagnostic test as certain benign diseases such as lymphomatoid papulosis, pityriasis lichenoides and cutaneous lymphoid hyperplasia may occasionally show such abnormalities.

Some illustrative examples

Case 1. A diagnostic biopsy from the trunk of a 36-year-old male with a long-standing, widespread, slightly pruritic, telangiectatic eruption. Low power (Figure 3.9a) shows a normal epidermis with basket-weave orthokeratosis. The superficial dermis shows mildly dilated capillaries with very slight hypercellularity.

This is a 'quiet' biopsy showing little obvious abnormality at low power. In this situation there is a list of disorders that need to be considered. Some of these are shown in Table 3.6. In this case, examination at high power (Figure 3.9b) with Giemsa staining shows an increase in perivascular mast cells with purple metachromatic granules.

Diagnosis: Urticaria pigmentosa (telangiectasia macularis eruptiva perstans variant).

Case 2. A diagnostic biopsy taken from a flat, pigmented lesion on the face of an elderly female. Low power (Figure 3.10a) shows normal epidermis on the left and an area of thickened epidermis to the right. The dermis appears normal. At higher power (Figure 3.10b)

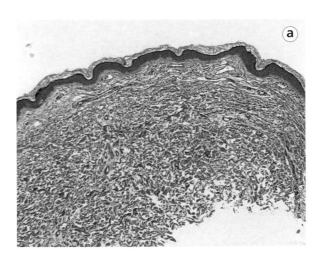
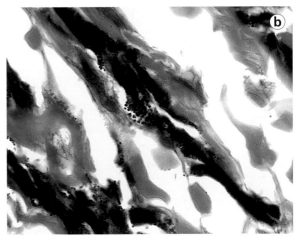

Figure 3.9
(a) Case 1. Low power magnification. (b) Case 1. High power (×100 — oil immersion). Giemsa stain.

43

Table 3.6: Some causes of a 'quiet' section with little or no obvious histological abnormality

Category	Features	Solution or further tests
Technical error	Too small a sample including normal skin only, or an immunofluorescence biopsy of normal skin sent for histology by mistake	Repeat the biopsy and take a larger specimen
Epidermal conditions:		
– ichthyoses	Compact hyperkeratosis	
– fungal infection	Patchy spongiosis and parakeratosis	PAS or Grocott stain
– porokeratosis	Cornoid lamellae easy to miss	Take more sections from block
– atrophic solar keratoses	May show little dysplasia	Ellipse biopsy to include normal skin for comparison
Dermal conditions:		
– urticaria	Slight oedema with a few inflammatory cells (especially eosinophils) around blood vessels	
– morphoea	Collagen bundles coarse, compact and hyalinized	Ellipse biopsy to include normal skin for comparison
– diffuse granuloma annulare	Collagen bundles dissected by mononuclear cells	
– anetoderma	Loss of elastic fibres	Elastic stain
– pseudoxanthoma elasticum	Dystrophic clumped elastic fibres	Elastic stain
– urticaria pigmentosa	Adult forms show fewer, rather dendritic mast cells	Chloroacetate esterase; Toluidine blue; Alcian blue
– blue naevi	Dendritic melanocytes in dermis	S-100 stain
– amyloid	Expanded dermal papillae may contain pink staining bodies	Congo red; Thioflavin T
– iron deposition		Perl's stain
– argyria	Silver granules seen near basement membrane of eccrine sweat glands	

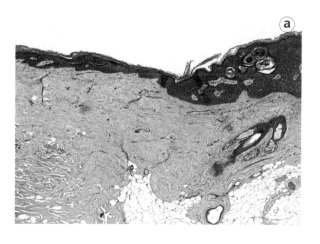 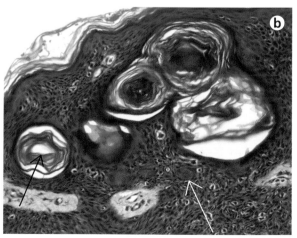

Figure 3.10

(a) Case 2. Low power. (b) Case 2. Higher power (×40). Detail of epidermal pathology. Black arrow: keratin inclusion cyst; white arrow: 'squamous eddy'.

the cellular detail in the thickened epidermis can be seen. The normal arrangement of the keratinocytes is disturbed with areas of 'stirred up' cells (squamous eddies) and small keratinous inclusion cysts (keratin pearls).

Diagnosis: Benign, non-inflamed seborrhoeic keratosis.

Case 3. A diagnostic biopsy from the flexural aspect of the wrist of a middle-aged female with an itchy papular eruption. Low power (×4) (Figure 3.11a) shows an upper dermal inflammatory infiltrate of mononuclear cells abutting the epidermis with some oedema. Vacuolar change is not prominent. The epidermis is not dysplastic but at higher power shows 'saw-toothing' of the rete ridges (black arrow) due to damage by the inflammatory process (Figure 3.11b).

This is an example of lichenoid interface dermatitis. The differential diagnosis includes lichen planus, lichenoid drug eruption and lichen striatus.

Diagnosis: Lichen planus.

Case 4. A diagnostic biopsy taken from the edge of an area of ulceration on the lower leg of an elderly male. Histology (×4) (Figure 3.12a) shows an area of crusted epidermal ulceration (blue arrow). The dermis contains islands of darkly staining tumour cells (white arrow) which show retraction artefact at the edge (black arrow). Examination at higher power (Figure 3.12b) shows the cells at the periphery of these islands to be aligned in rows (palisaded).

This is an example of 'blue balls in the dermis' for which there is a very wide differential diagnosis including primary and secondary skin tumours of many types. Sometimes it is necessary to carry out special cell marker studies to clarify the diagnosis. In clinical practice the most common diagnosis is basal cell carcinoma.

Diagnosis: Basal cell carcinoma.

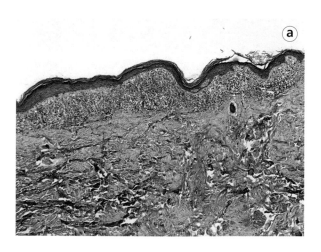 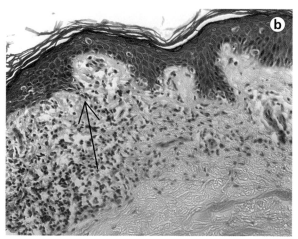

Figure 3.11
(a) Case 3. Low power (×4). (b) Case 3. High power (×40). Black arrow: 'saw-toothing' of epidermis.

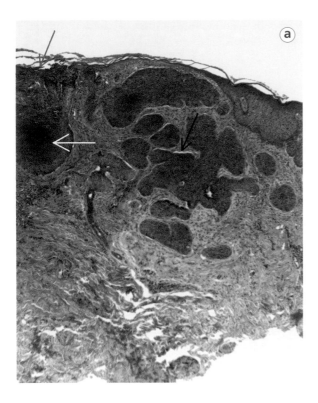

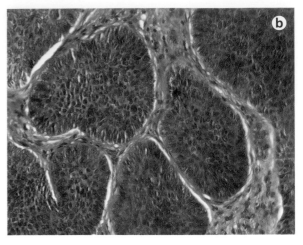

Figure 3.12
(a) Case 4. Low power (×4). (b) Case 4. High power (×40).

CONCLUSION

As an intermediate step in learning histopathology, it is recommended to try to develop a visual correlation between the clinical and histopathological appearance of skin conditions. This can be done by studying one of a number of dermatological atlases that include histology such as the latest edition of Du Vivier's atlas. There are many excellent full reference texts on dermatopathology and any serious student of dermatology should invest in such a book at an early stage of their career (*see* Further reading).

Finally, there is no substitute for practice:

• Look regularly at the slides of your own cases.
• Study the 'teaching slides' in your teaching hospital.
• Attend meetings with your histopathologists.

References

1. Cerio R, Calonje E. Histopathology of the skin: general principles. In: Burns T, Breathnach S, Cox N, Griffiths CEM, eds. Rook's textbook of dermatology. 7th edn. Oxford: Blackwell Science; 2004:7.1–7.44.

2. Michel B, Milner Y, David K. Preservation of fixed tissue immunoglobulins in skin biopsies of patients with lupus erythematosus and bullous diseases: preliminary report. J Invest Dermatol 1973; 59:449–452.

3. Mondragon G, Nygaard F. Routine and special procedures for processing biopsy specimens of lesions suspected to be malignant melanomas. Am J Dermatopathol 1981; 3:265–272.

4. Bancroft JD, Stevens A, eds. Theory and practice of histological techniques. 3rd edn. Edinburgh: Churchill Livingstone; 1990.

5. Ackerman AB. Histologic diagnosis of inflammatory skin diseases. Philadelphia: Lea and Febiger; 1978.

6. Wallace ML, Smoller BR. Immunohistochemistry and diagnostic dermatopathology. J Am Acad Dermatol 1996; 34:163–183.

7. Momose H, Mehta P, Battifora H. Antigen retrieval by microwave irradiation in lead thiocyanate. Comparison with protease-digestion retrieval. Appl Immunohistochem 1993; 1:77–82.

8. Kelly SE, Wojnarowska F. The use of chemically split tissue in the detection of circulating anti-basement zone antibodies in bullous pemphigoid and cicatricial pemphigoid. Br J Dermatol 1988; 117:31–40.

9. Schaumberg-Lever, G. Immunoenzyme techniques in dermatopathology. Int J Dermatol 1986; 25:217–223.

10. Schach CP, Smoller BR, Hudson AR. Immunohistochemical stains in dermatopathology. J Am Acad Dermatol 2000; 43:1094–1100.

11. His ED, Yegappan S. Lymphoma immunophenotyping: a new era in paraffin-section immunohistochemistry. Adv Anat Pathol 2001; 8:218–239.

12. Rees JL. Molecular biology. In: Burns T, Breathnach S, Cox N, Griffiths CEM, eds. Rook's textbook of dermatology. 7th edn. Oxford: Blackwell Science; 2004:8.1–8.24

13. Wood GS. Molecular biologic techniques for the diagnosis of cutaneous lymphomas. In: Barnhill RL, ed. Textbook of dermatopathology. New York: McGraw-Hill; 1998:864–869.

Further reading

Ackerman AB. Histologic diagnosis of inflammatory skin diseases. Philadelphia: Lippincott-Williams and Wilkins; 1978.

Barnhill RL, ed. Textbook of dermatopathology. New York: McGraw-Hill; 1998.

Du Vivier, A. Atlas of clinical dermatology. 3rd edn. Edinburgh: Churchill Livingstone; 2002.

Elder D, Elenitsas R, Johnson B Jr, Murphy G, eds. Lever's histopathology of the skin. 9th edn. Philadelphia: Lippincott; 2005.

MacDonald D, Ben-Gashir M, Robson A. Dermatopathology. Oxford: Blackwell; 2005.

McKee PH, Calonje E, Granter S. Pathology of the skin. 3rd edn. Philadelphia: Lippincott; 2005.

Weedon D, Strutton G. Skin pathology. 2nd edn. Edinburgh: Churchill Livingstone; 2002.

Inflammatory skin diseases

4

Victoria J. Lewis and Andrew Y. Finlay

INTRODUCTION

The diagnosis and management of patients with inflammatory skin disease remains a very challenging and rewarding aspect of 'core' dermatology practice. Thorough history taking and examination, sometimes aided by histopathology, remain at the heart of good management. Skills in the management of chronic disease need to be developed, such as the ability to communicate risk/benefit of different therapy strategies and reach joint decisions with patients. You should try to understand the impact of the disease on the patients' lives.

It is important to become familiar with current published national guidelines in the UK, published by the British Association of Dermatologists (website http://www.bad.org.uk). New topical and systemic therapies are being developed and marketed specifically for psoriasis; remember to take an appropriate cautious approach to new therapies. Over the last 30 years many new drugs have been introduced with much optimism and marketed extensively only to be dropped because of poor effectiveness or side effects; you need to take a long term perspective with your patients who have long term disease.

PSORIASIS

Epidemiology

Two percent of the World's population suffer from psoriasis vulgaris. Countries further from the equator have higher prevalence rates (Northern Europe and North America — up to 4.8%; Africa and Asia — < 1%). Psoriasis can first appear from infancy to the eighth decade, and there is a bimodal onset peak.

- Late teens/early 20s — Often more severe, and with a positive family history.
- 50–60 years.

It affects males and females equally, but onset is often earlier in females.

Aetiology

Psoriasis is thought to arise from an environmental trigger, on top of a genetic susceptibility.

Genetic susceptibility

In psoriasis, the genetics are complex and polygenic. Evidence for genetic factors has been formed from family and twin studies, showing increased concordance in both dizygotic and monozygotic twins. Much work has been done on HLA linkage and genetic loci.

The most important identified so far are:

- HLA Cw6 — strongest association with severe disease of early onset.
- PSORS1 gene (chromosome 6p21.3).

Environmental triggers

- Trauma: Koebner phenomenon — occurrence of psoriasis in an area of trauma or a scar. (Box 4.1 and Figure 4.1)
- Infection: Streptococcal throat infection has a strong association with acute guttate psoriasis (Figure 4.1), and also an important association with chronic plaque psoriasis. HIV infection can make psoriasis worse. This is paradoxical and unexplained — one would expect a T-cell mediated disease such as psoriasis to improve with T-cell depletion.

Box 4.1: Skin conditions which commonly display Koebner phenomenon

- Psoriasis
- Lichen planus
- Viral warts
- Vitiligo

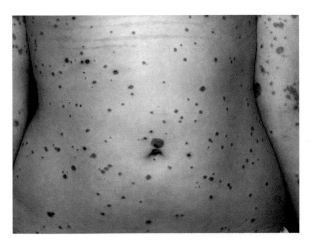

Figure 4.1
Guttate psoriasis. Note the small widespread scaly plaques on arms and torso. Also note the 'Koebner phenomenon' — psoriasis plaques at the umbilicus due to the trauma of 'belly button' piercing.

- Drugs: Some drugs can precipitate or worsen psoriasis (Box 4.2).
- Sunlight: Most patients' psoriasis improves in the sun, but some (about 10%) get worse.
- Metabolic: Pregnancy generally improves psoriasis, but it can worsen post-partum. Generalized pustular psoriasis can be triggered post-partum, or by hypocalcaemia.
- Stress: There is strong evidence that stress can exacerbate psoriasis. Patients with high levels of worry respond less well to therapy.
- Alcohol: Heavy consumption can worsen existing disease.
- Smoking: There is a strong link between smoking and palmoplantar pustular psoriasis, particularly in females.

Pathogenesis

The three main features are:

1. Epidermal proliferation and loss of differentiation — clinically causing scaling and thickening.
2. Dilatation and proliferation of dermal blood vessels — clinically causing erythema.
3. Accumulation of inflammatory cells, mainly neutrophils and T-lymphocytes.

The T-lymphocyte

Psoriasis is a T-cell mediated disease. Th1 helper cells predominate, which, when activated, secrete TNF-α, IL-3, IL-6, GM-CSF and IFN-γ.

TNF-α is the most important and has direct therapy relevance (Table 4.1). IL-8 and IL-10 may have future direct therapy relevance.

Clinical features of chronic plaque psoriasis

- Sharply demarcated, erythematous, papulosquamous plaques occur, mainly on the extensor surfaces (Figure 4.2). They can vary in size from < 1 mm to > 20 cm, and are covered in silvery-white scale, which, when scratched off, may cause pinpoint bleeding. This is known as the 'Auspitz sign', which is *not* recommended to be used. When covered with emollient the plaques will instantly appear more red.
- Erythema at the edge of the plaque indicates active psoriasis, and is useful to assess response to therapy. Post-inflammatory hypo- or hyperpigmentation can occur.

Box 4.2: Drugs which can precipitate or worsen psoriasis

- Lithium
- Beta-blockers
- Withdrawal of corticosteroids
- Non-steroidal anti-inflammatory drugs
- Antimalarials
- ACE inhibitors

Table 4.1: Management of psoriasis

Therapy	Top tips
Bath additives/soap substitutes/emollients	All essential. See Table 4.3 for further details
Topical vitamin D analogues	First line treatment. Can use in combination with topical steroids for limited periods. Some preparations can irritate sensitive areas of skin
Topical corticosteroids	Often first choice for sensitive areas of skin. Potent steroid use or withdrawal can lead to a rebound flare of psoriasis, or transformation to generalized pustular psoriasis
Topical coal tar	Some preparations are messy and smelly. Particularly good for small plaque/guttate psoriasis (apply to all of skin) or scalp
Topical dithranol (anthralin)	Works well on thick plaques. Started at a low concentration and built up. Apply to plaques only. Can irritate surrounding skin. Causes staining of skin
UVB	Main complications burning and skin cancer risk. Patient consent required before commencing. Starting dose determined by Minimum Erythema Dose. Maximum permitted lifetime dose
PUVA	Psoralen can be oral or topical (bath, gel, paint). If taking oral preparation need to protect eyes from UVA for 24 hours (UVA opaque glasses)
Systemics: acitretin methotrexate ciclosporin mycophenolate mofetil	See Chapter 7
The 'biologics'	These are antibodies or receptor blockers to TNF-α. All require intravenous or subcutaneous administration, and multiple doses. The main problems are increased risk of infections, particularly reactivation of tuberculosis, antibody formation, and the expense of the drug. See Chapter 7

Diagnosis

The diagnosis of psoriasis is usually straightforward, but confusion can arise in flexural psoriasis, scalp psoriasis and palmoplantar psoriasis.

Flexural psoriasis

There are some patients who present with indistinct inflammatory lesions in the flexural areas who have inflamed skin at some typical psoriatic sites (always check for psoriasis at the umbilicus in this case), but who also have involvement at sites typical of seborrhoeic dermatitis. The groin area, vulva, axilla, submammary cleft and gluteal cleft can be affected, again with minimal scale, also causing some diagnostic confusion with intertrigo (the two can co-exist). This so-called 'sebo-psoriasis' may need to be treated with a combination of topical antifungals, topical steroids and then standard psoriasis therapies. Do not be worried if this presentation leaves you feeling not sure of the diagnosis — it can be very difficult. A biopsy is usually not helpful as mixed inflammatory features are seen.

51

Figure 4.2
Chronic plaque psoriasis. Note the thickened plaque on the knee topped with heavy scaling.

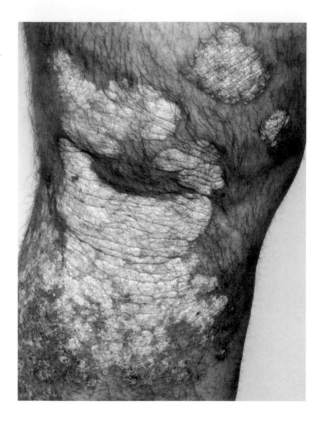

Scalp psoriasis

Scalp psoriasis is usually easy to diagnose; there are typical lesions elsewhere and the lesions are very clearly defined. Plaques on the scalp can develop severe adherent scaling, termed pityriasis amiantacea. Hair growth is usually normal unless severely affected. Occasionally you will see patients misdiagnosed as having scalp psoriasis, even though they have the typical diffuse changes of seborrhoeic dermatitis and no evidence of psoriasis elsewhere. Remember the value of topical antifungals in this setting. Generally, topical coal tar preparations or corticosteroid preparations are used for this condition.

Palmoplantar pustular psoriasis (Figure 4.3)

Psoriasis of the palms or soles can sometimes be difficult to differentiate from chronic eczema. Look carefully for vesicles — these clear sago-like small blebs are diagnostic of eczema. A mixture of large fresh yellow and older brown pustules are typical of palmoplantar pustular psoriasis, but in eczema, vesicles can sometimes get infected, also producing pustules, but no typical burnt-out older brown areas. This is a difficult condition to treat, and potent topical corticosteroids, localized PUVA, or oral retinoids are standard treatments for this condition.

Assessment of disease severity

The reality of most consultations with psoriasis patients is that severity is based on the patient's and clinician's overall view as to whether the disease is getting better or worse.

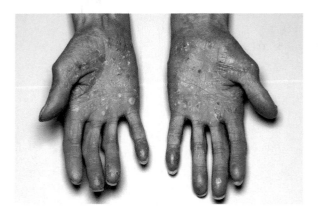

Figure 4.3
Palmar pustular psoriasis. Note the different colours of the pustules indicating different maturity of lesions.

You should, however, know about some basic ways to assess psoriasis severity: these include body surface area estimation (BSA), the PASI (psoriasis area and severity index) scoring system[1] and methods to measure the impact of psoriasis on life quality, e.g. the psoriasis disability index (PDI)[2] or the DLQI (dermatology life quality index).[3]

Body surface area estimation

Use the handprint method. The area of the full palmar aspect of one hand, including the palm and the five digits, is approximately equal to 1% body surface area. It is possible to very quickly estimate BSA by this method, imagining roughly how smaller areas would coalesce into one handprint.

PASI

In this method, an estimate of the severity of redness, scaling and thickness is made in each of the four areas: head, upper limbs, trunk and lower limbs. An estimate of the area involved within each of these areas is also made and the results calculated in a formula, resulting in a score from 0 (no involvement) to 72 (worst possible involvement). A summary of the PASI formula is given in Table 4.2.

DLQI

This is a simple 10 question standard validated questionnaire which can be used across all skin diseases, including psoriasis, to measure the adverse impact of the disease on the patient's life. It takes about 2 minutes to complete and gives a score from 0 (no impact) to 30 (maximum possible impact). The score can be easily interpreted thus: 0–1 = no impact, 2–5 = slight impact, 6–10 = moderate impact, 11–20 = very great impact, 21–30 = extremely great impact. More information is available on www.dlqi.com, or www.dermatology.org.uk.[4]

We have suggested that current severe psoriasis can be defined by the Rule of Tens: BSA > 10% *or* PASI > 10 *or* DLQI > 10.

Variants of psoriasis

Ten percent of all psoriasis sufferers have a variant of the condition.

Pustular psoriasis

Sheets of small, sterile pustules can appear in plaques of otherwise normal-appearing skin. When generalized, the patient can be systemically unwell, and this represents a dermatological emergency. This can appear post-partum, with hypocalcaemia, as a rebound to withdrawal of topical or systemic steroids, or following infection. Oral methotrexate is often the first line treatment for control of this condition.

Nail psoriasis

Nail changes are seen in 25–50% of psoriasis sufferers (Figure 4.4). These include pitting, ridging and discoloration of the nail, subungual hyperkeratosis, onycholysis and a circular 'oil spot' appearance (due to hyperkeratosis of the nail bed).

Table 4.2: Formula for calculation of PASI score

Score	0	1	2	3	4	5	6
Erythema Induration Scaling	none	slight	moderate	severe	very severe		
Area %	0	1–9	10–29	30–49	50–69	70–89	90–100

	Head (H)	Upper limbs (U)	Trunk (T)	Lower limbs (L)
Erythema (E)	–	–	–	–
Induration (I)	–	–	–	–
Scaling (S)	–	–	–	–
Sum = E + I + S =	__	__	__	__
Area	–	–	–	–
Sum × Area =	__	__	__	__
	× 0.1	× 0.2	× 0.3	× 0.4
Total =	__.__	__.__	__.__	__.__

PASI score = Total (H) + Total (T) + Total (U) + Total (L) = __.__

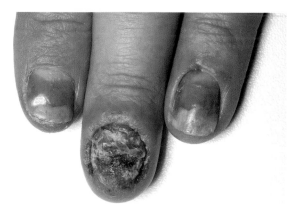

Figure 4.4
Psoriasis of nails. Note the onycholysis and nail pitting.

Acrodermatitis of Hallopeau

There are painful pustules on the tips of the fingers and under the nail bed, often with shedding of the nail plate.

Psoriatic arthritis

It is reported that 5–30% of patients with psoriasis also suffer from a form of arthritis. This can be:

- Mono/asymmetrical arthritis.
- Distal interphalangeal joint involvement — associated with nail involvement.
- Rheumatoid arthritis-like pattern.
- Arthritis mutilans.
- Spondylitis/sacroiliitis — increased in HLA B27 haplotypes.

Management of chronic plaque psoriasis

All dermatology textbooks list the various options for treating psoriasis, but few address the reality of the decision-making process. This is a complicated matter involving education of and negotiation with the patient. Flow charts are usually inadequate to describe the process, which is heavily influenced by the individual patient's previous experience of different therapies, their attitudes towards risk, the practicalities of using topical therapy and the current impact that the disease is having on the patient's life.

Table 4.1 shows the main topical and systemic treatments used for this condition. Management of psoriasis variants is covered under the individual sections. The Psoriasis Association is a useful point of contact and information for patients.[5]

ECZEMA

Eczema, or dermatitis (these are interchangeable terms), is an inflammatory skin reaction, featuring itching, redness, scaling and clustered papulovesicles. Eczema can be endogenous (from within the body) or exogenous (from an external trigger). Boxes 4.3 and 4.4 show the main subtypes of this.

ATOPIC DERMATITIS

Epidemiology

Atopic dermatitis has a prevalence of 10–20%, the highest prevalence being in the most developed Westernized countries. Immigrant populations, e.g. black Afro-Caribbean children residing in London, have twice the prevalence of atopic eczema of their Caucasian counterparts. Ninety percent of cases begin before the age of 5 years. The prevalence of atopic diseases in general, and atopic eczema in particular, has been increasing over the last four decades.

Diagnosis

This is made according to the UK Working Party's refinement of Hanifin and Rajka's diagnostic criteria for atopic dermatitis (Box 4.5).[6] Unlike most disease criteria, this set has been validated.

Aetiology

Atopic eczema is thought to arise from an interaction of genetic and environmental factors.

Box 4.3: *Types/causes of exogenous eczema*

- Irritant contact dermatitis
- Allergic contact dermatitis
- Photoallergic/photoaggravated dermatitis
- Infective (secondary to bacterial/viral/fungal infection)
- Post-traumatic (rare, and NOT Koebner phenomenon)

Box 4.4: *Types of endogenous eczema*

- Atopic dermatitis
- Seborrhoeic dermatitis
- Asteatotic eczema
- Discoid eczema
- Hand eczema
- Gravitational/varicose eczema
- Eczematous drug eruptions
- Lichen simplex

Box 4.5: *Criteria for diagnosis of atopic dermatitis*[6]

The child must have an itchy skin condition (or parental report of scratching or rubbing in a child).

Plus three or more of the following:

1. Onset below age 2 years (not used if child is under 4 years)
2. History of skin crease involvement (including cheeks in children under 10 years)
3. History of generally dry skin
4. Personal history of other atopic disease (or history of any atopic disease in a first degree relative in children under 4 years)
5. Visible flexural dermatitis (or dermatitis of cheeks/forehead and outer limbs in children under 4 years)

Genetic and intrauterine factors

Parental (particularly maternal) history of atopy is one of the strongest risk factors for the development of atopy. Also, a higher birth weight correlates with increasing prevalence of atopic eczema.

Environmental factors

- *Pollution* — indoor (e.g. cigarette smoke) and outdoor (e.g. industrial) pollutants may increase the prevalence of atopic eczema.
- *The hygiene hypothesis* — children from large families, and those living in the developing world, have lower prevalence of atopic eczema. This may be due to early exposure to microbes, particularly those causing faeco-oral infection, thus driving the immune system to a protective response.
- *The home environment* — in moderate to severe eczema, reduction of house dust mite levels in the home may be of benefit. The main advice to give would be:
  - Frequent vacuuming of carpets or avoidance of carpets if possible.
  - Frequent dusting and ventilation of bedroom, and vacuuming of mattress every week.
  - Covering bedding with dust tight mattress and pillow covers.
  - Frequent washing of soft toys, or putting them in the freezer for 24 hours.

Other points of advice for the home would be:

- Avoidance of animal dander.
- Wearing of cotton clothes rather than wool.
- Washing clothes in non-fragranced, non-bio detergents, at higher temperatures (> 50°C).

Food

Food allergy can potentially aggravate atopic eczema in children less than one year old. Over the age of one its role is much less clear, and more unlikely. The best advice, if parents insist on following the dietary route, is to eliminate a certain food from the diet, singly, for 6 weeks only, to determine the effect of its avoidance (in the case of milk avoidance ensure other sources of calcium are given). The involvement of a dietician may be helpful to advise on safe and appropriate dietary manipulation. RAST (radioallergosorbent test) blood tests are available to diagnose food allergy, but the relationship between these antibodies in the blood and the effect on the skin is not predictable, thus the test is not a reliable basis for practical advice, and is best avoided.

Immunology

Patients with eczema have dry skin, with disruption of the epidermal barrier, increased transepidermal water loss, and increased entry of environmental allergens, so inducing the Th2-dominant immune response.

The Th1/Th2 response

T-helper cells, in their development, differentiate into Th1 cells (secrete cytokines IL-2 and IFN-α), or Th2 cells (secrete cytokines IL-4, IL-5 and IL-13). Which helper cell they become depends on what signals they receive externally. In eczema, Th2 cells are mainly produced, secreting IL-4, and IL-5, which stimulate B-cells to produce more IgE, the main immunoglobulin involved in the pathogenesis of atopic disease.

Clinical features (Figure 4.5)

These include:

- Itching.
- Dry skin.
- Erythematous macules, papules or papulovesicles.
- Crusting.
- Excoriation and lichenification.
- Secondary infection.

Distribution

This often varies with age.

Infantile — usually most severe on the face (especially if excessive drooling is present). When crawling, extensor surfaces can become rubbed and affected by eczema.

Childhood (from 18 months to 2 years) — mainly affecting elbow and knee flexures, neck, wrists and ankles. The neck can show fine pigmentation, a 'dirty neck'. In Asian or Black skin, extensor distribution of the eczema is more common.

Adult — the eczema has a similar distribution to that of children, often with lichenified areas.

The course of atopic eczema

In 90% of affected children, the eczema starts before the age of 5 years. It tends to run a course of remissions and exacerbations. There is a general tendency towards spontaneous improvement throughout childhood. Clearance occurs in 50% by the age of 13 years. Severe persistent adult atopic eczema is seen, but is much less common than childhood eczema.

Figure 4.5
Atopic eczema. Note the flexural erythema, lichenification and secondary infection of the skin.

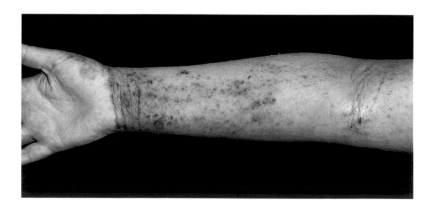

Complications

Bacterial infection: this is secondary, and is often streptococcal or staphylococcal, mainly *Staphylococcus aureus*.

Viral infection:

a) secondary infection with herpes simplex virus can cause 'eczema herpeticum' (Figures 4.6 and 4.7). This is a *dermatological emergency*. There is sudden onset of numerous painful small fluid-filled vesicles. This can become secondarily impetiginized, can cause systemic upset, and can also affect the conjunctivae. Systemic antivirals are indicated (oral is usually adequate), and topical corticosteroids or immunosuppressants should be stopped;

b) there is increased spread of viral warts and molluscum contagiosum. However, varicella zoster virus affects eczema sufferers in the same way as it would those with normal skin.

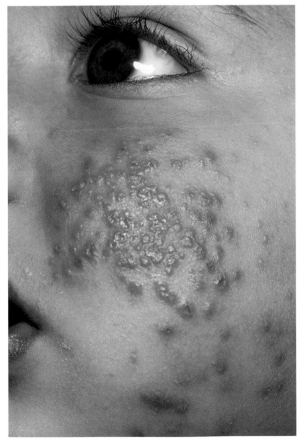

Figure 4.6
Eczema herpeticum (early). Note the tiny numerous fluid-filled blisters on the cheek.

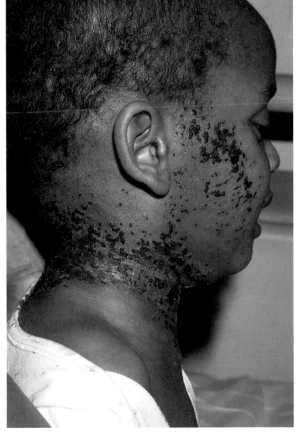

Figure 4.7
Eczema herpeticum (late). No blisters remain but there are tiny discrete erosions and secondary bacterial infection and crusting on the cheek and neck.

Ocular abnormalities: These include conjunctival irritation, keratoconus (a conical cornea leading to marked visual disturbance which is rare), and cataract (mainly if severe facial eczema, or use of strong topical or systemic corticosteroids).

Measurement of severity of eczema

This can be measured physically, for example, by the Eczema Assessment and Severity Index[7] or SCORAD.[8] It is also important to ask about the effect of eczema on quality of life, either with specific measures, such as the Dermatology Life Quality Index[3,4] or Children's Dermatology Life Quality Index,[4,9] or by general enquiry about itch, sleep loss, and loss of time at work. In children, their growth and progress at school should be particularly noted. All of these factors should influence decisions regarding management.

Treatment

As with any chronic inflammatory condition of the skin, time should be taken to develop a good relationship between the dermatologist and the patient, particularly in increasing understanding about the nature and course of the disease. Management should be based on a specific overall regimen, including bath additives, soap substitutes, emollients, and topical steroids or topical immunosuppressants.

This maintenance regimen should be *written down* for the patient. A second regimen specifically for flare-ups should also be *written down* for them, also specifying when they can go back to their usual treatments. Quantity of topical treatments required should be discussed and, if possible, demonstrated during the consultation. Treatment concordance is the biggest problem to tackle, and any reluctance to use the prescribed medication should be discussed (e.g. treatments which sting, fear about side effects of topical steroids, reluctance to ask GP for repeat prescriptions). This all takes time but is well worth it in the long term. Always inform the patient or parents about the National Eczema Society which is an excellent source of information.[10]

A summary of specific treatments is included in Table 4.3.

My patient is not improving with conventional eczema treatment

If eczema fails to improve with correct treatment, or worsens, the following should be considered:

Is the diagnosis correct?

Other differential diagnoses

- Scabies: Always look for scabies burrows, particularly on the finger webs, abdomen and genital area.
- Seborrhoeic dermatitis: This mainly affects the scalp, eyebrows and creases on the face. Greasy scales are clinically visible.

Table 4.3: *Management of atopic dermatitis*

Therapy	Top tips
Bath and shower additives	All patients should have one of these and be advised to avoid soaps, bubble bath and shower gels. Some contain antiseptic, important if the patient has recurrent infections. Care must be taken as some make the bath or shower very slippery.
Soap substitutes	Most emollients can also be used as soap substitutes.
Emollients	These are essential and should be applied liberally. They vary in intensity. Stick with one that the patient likes and tolerates, and is willing to use, to improve concordance.
Topical corticosteroids	These come in a range of potencies, and a 'step-up' and 'step-down' regimen can be used according to severity of eczema. More potent corticosteroids should be used for palms and soles, and less potent drugs for the face and neck. Some contain antibiotics and/or antifungals. These are useful in flexural areas, but antibiotic resistance can develop.
Topical immunomodulators Tacrolimus Pimecrolimus	These are steroid sparing, so useful particularly on the face or neck, or where the patient required potent topical steroids for long periods. These should be applied intermittently, beginning at the first signs of a new flare. They may feel 'burning' for the first few days of application. Due to lack of long term data on skin cancer risk, sun protection information should be given for patients specifically on these drugs.
UVB	As for Table 4.1.
Systemic treatments: Ciclosporin Azathioprine	See Chapter 7.

Is there an element of irritant contact dermatitis?

Atopic dermatitis patients are more prone to this, particularly on the hands.

Is there an allergic contact dermatitis?

Eczema in localized sites, e.g. the face or hands, or eczema which is unresponsive or worsening, may indicate an allergic contact dermatitis. Patients with atopic dermatitis are more prone to contact allergy. Also they are more likely to become sensitized to fragrances, topical steroids or preservatives in their treatments. Patch testing is indicated if this is suspected (see Chapter 6).

ACNE

Acne is a chronic inflammatory disorder of the pilosebaceous units. A pilosebaceous unit consists of a hair follicle, erector pili muscle, sebaceous gland, and associated apocrine and eccrine sweat glands.

Epidemiology of acne

Acne usually starts in adolescence and mainly resolves by the mid-twenties, although 10–20% of cases persist into adulthood, particularly females. Almost half of male and female adolescents develop acne to varying degrees, 10% of whom have severe acne. The peak prevalence is 14–16 years for females, and 16–19 years in males, reflecting earlier onset of puberty in females.

What if my patient has atypical features?

In patients who present at a younger age, or have more severe, refractory acne, the following should be considered and investigated as necessary:

- Precocious puberty.
- Polycystic ovarian syndrome.
- Hyperandrogenism.
- Hypercortisolism (including Cushing's syndrome).
- XYY chromosomal phenotype.

Acne can have some additional external causes which should be considered and enquired about in patients with atypical or refractory acne:

- Premenstrual flaring of acne: This type of acne responds best to hormonal modulation (see Table 4.4).
- Occupation: Patients dealing with heavy-duty oils and crude tars in their work are more susceptible. Those working with chlorinated hydrocarbons, if accidentally released, may develop chloracne which is relatively resistant to treatment and may take several years to resolve.
- Physical factors: Certain cosmetics, particularly those with an oily base, are comedogenic. Pomades, which are used to defrizz curly Afro-Caribbean hair, also have a comedogenic effect.
- Drugs: The commonest acne-inducing drugs are anabolic steroids, corticosteroids, phenytoin, lithium, isoniazid and iodides. It is important to ask about prescription and non-prescription drugs.

Pathogenesis

Acne appears to occur due to:

- Increased sebum production: this is mainly dependent on androgenic sex hormones of gonadal or adrenal origin.
- Genetically inherited distribution of sebaceous glands: increased numbers and size of glands appear to have a strong familial tendency, particularly in severe acne. Genetics are thought to be multifactorial.
- Hypercornification of the pilosebaceous duct, forming micro-comedones: comedones are due to abnormalities in proliferation and differentiation of ductal keratinocytes. Several

Table 4.4: Management of acne

Therapy	Top tips
Topical benzoyl peroxide Topical azelaic acid	All topical treatments for acne can irritate or dry the skin. Benzoyl peroxide can bleach clothes/bedclothes. Antimicrobial.
Topical retinoids	For oily skin, gels are often better to dry the skin. Topical retinoids contraindicated in pregnancy. Anticomedonal.
Topical antibiotics in combination with benzoyl peroxide/zinc	Some preparations can glow under ultraviolet strobe lights. Antibiotic resistance can occur.
Oral antibiotics Tetracyclines	At least 6 months of treatment should be given. Contraindicated in pregnancy and young children. Minocycline can cause blue-black pigmentation, more likely if higher dose for long duration of therapy; also avoid if history/family history of SLE as can cause a lupus-like syndrome.
Erythromycin Trimethoprim	Dose 500 mg BD. High dose 300 mg BD as second line treatment.
Hormonal treatments Cyproterone acetate Spironolactone	Oral contraceptive, suppresses sebum production. Particularly useful for premenstrual flare of acne, or for acne related to polycystic ovarian syndrome.
Isotretinoin	Most common side effects are dryness of lips, skin and mucous membranes. Hair thinning and nosebleeds are also not uncommon. Depression and suicide risk is still unclear –– ask about personal or family history of depression before starting treatment.
Blue light/blue-red light treatments	Small trials have shown moderate improvement.
Laser treatment	Small trials have shown moderate improvement with NLite laser treatment. This is not usually available on the NHS, and is contraindicated in patients on photosensitizing drugs, or on isotretinoin, due to risk of scarring.
Physical treatments Cryotherapy Intralesional triamcinolone Cautery	This can be used for old acne nodules. This can be helpful for acne keloid scars, and for early acne nodules. Closed comedones respond well to this.
Treatments of acne scarring	These are usually not available on the NHS. They comprise of: Excision of scars Dermabrasion Laser resurfacing Chemical peeling Collagen injection

factors are involved in this, including sebaceous lipid composition, bacteria, local cytokine production and androgens.

- Abnormality of microbial flora, especially *Propionibacterium acnes*: patients with acne have more *P. acnes* on their skin, but levels do not correspond to clinical severity. The bacteria may induce inflammation.
- Production of inflammation: this is partly due to duct rupture, bacterial colonization and hormonal factors.

Clinical features (Figures 4.8 and 4.9)

The main features are:

- Seborrhoea.
- Open and closed comedones — 'blackheads' and 'whiteheads'.
- Erythematous papules.
- Nodules.
- Deep pustules.
- Pseudocysts.
- Scarring.

How to assess the severity of acne

Acne should be assessed both in physical terms, and in terms of its effect on the individual, in order to decide on the best management options for the patient. The most frequently used measure of physical severity for research purposes is the Leeds acne grading system.[11]

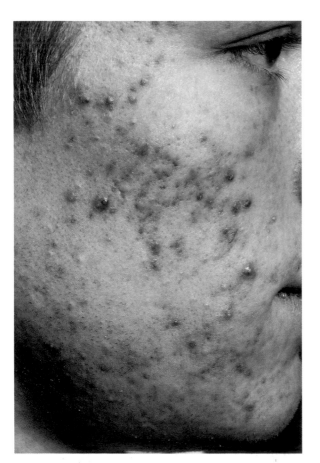

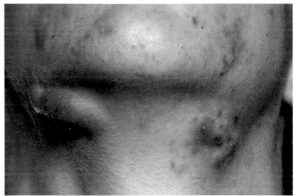

Figure 4.9
Severe nodulocystic acne. Note the open and closed comedones, cysts and keloid scarring under the chin (this should not be surgically excised).

Figure 4.8
Moderate/severe acne. Note the papules, pustules, comedones and mild scarring on the cheek.

However, this scale was developed before the introduction of isotretinoin and is biased towards extremely severe acne. It is useful to have a descriptive record of areas involved and presence/absence of cysts/scars/pustules/papules.

The psychological and social effects of acne cannot be underestimated. Often it comes on in adolescence, a time where embarrassment and lack of confidence are highest. Social contact may become limited, bullying may occur at school, and it may even have an effect on employment prospects. It is important to have some of idea of what the patient is going through, even in an outpatient consultation. More formal measures of quality of life can be used, such as the Dermatology Life Quality Index,[3,4] or an acne specific measure such as the Cardiff Acne Disability Index or the Acne Quality of Life Scale.[4]

Differential diagnosis

The main alternative diagnoses to consider would be:

- Rosacea. Typically, there are *no comedones* in rosacea.
- Perioral dermatitis. There is often a history of topical steroid use in the perioral area.
- Folliculitis. Gram-negative organisms, *Pityrosporum* and *Demodex* mite can cause a folliculitis, which may present as acne refractory to treatment. A trial of topical antibiotic, anti-yeast preparation, or permethrin, can help to differentiate between these.

Management

When managing a patient with acne, it is firstly important to address any misconceptions about what has caused it, for example:

- Diet: Many patients still believe that eating fats or chocolate can cause acne. There is no convincing evidence to suggest that diet plays any part in acne development.
- Lack of hygiene: Again, patients believe that 'blackheads' are due to dirt, and use abrasive or irritating preparations to cleanse their skin excessively. It is important to explain that the 'black' in a 'blackhead' is pigment, not dirt, and that excessive cleansing of the skin with these chemicals can make acne worse, as well as irritating the skin, causing dryness and soreness. A bland, non-irritating preparation, or just water, should be used to wash the skin.
- Make-up: As mentioned previously, there is some truth that greasy make-ups can cause acne. It is important to recommend a non-comedogenic formulation of make-up, and also recommend that it is completely removed before going to sleep at night. It is unrealistic to expect adolescent girls to go without make-up so a compromise should be reached on this.

Table 4.4 outlines the specific treatments used for acne.

How to treat a patient safely with isotretinoin

Isotretinoin is a very effective drug for severe, scarring, or non-responsive acne. However, it has many side effects, some of which are serious, and the benefits and risks of this treatment should be carefully weighed up before commencing the course. The following section describes current guidelines for the use of isotretinoin, but always consult the British Association of Dermatologists website for the most up-to-date guidelines.[12]

At first consultation, a written Medicines and Healthcare products Regulatory Agency (MHRA) approved patient information booklet should be given to the patient, and the main side effects (particularly the possible link with depression), indications and course of treatment discussed. It is useful to record any personal or family history of depression at this stage. Isotretinoin is *teratogenic* and any female considered for treatment with this drug should be assessed for their potential risk of pregnancy. All should be issued with a contraception information booklet, and sign to acknowledge their receipt of this. Baseline screening blood tests (including liver function tests and fasting lipids) should also be performed at this stage.

At a second consultation, provided the patient would like to go ahead with treatment, and all baseline blood tests are normal, the male patient can receive their full course of isotretinoin. All other topical acne treatments and systemic antibiotics should be stopped. Any female considered at risk of pregnancy will then be part of the pregnancy prevention plan.

Pregnancy prevention plan

Prescriber, pharmacist and patients must follow these rules:

- Pregnancy test just before starting therapy. Pregnancy tests can be from blood or urine but must be medically supervised. Isotretinoin should be started on the second day of the next period.
- One and preferably two forms of contraception to be used from at least 1 month before until at least 1 month after course of isotretinoin.
- Monthly pregnancy tests throughout therapy.
- Pregnancy test 5 weeks after stopping course of therapy.
- Isotretinoin prescriptions — for only 1 month of therapy at a time. Prescriptions are valid for 7 days only.
- Complete the checklist for prescribing to female patients at each stage, i.e. pre-treatment, each in-treatment visit and post-treatment visit.

If the patient is not regarded as at risk of pregnancy, and does not enter the pregnancy prevention plan, the reason for this should be recorded in the notes.

What if my patient becomes pregnant while on isotretinoin?

If pregnancy occurs or is suspected in any female patient during treatment or in the 5 weeks after therapy:

Patient should stop isotretinoin treatment immediately.
Patient should receive advice from a physician specialized or experienced in birth defects.
Patient should inform the primary prescriber of isotretinoin and the GP.
The supplier and the MHRA should be informed if pregnancy is confirmed.

How much isotretinoin can I give?

The standard dose of isotretinoin in the UK is up to 1 mg/kg/day for 16 weeks, and a single treatment course is sufficient for the majority of patients. A further improvement of acne can be observed up to 8 weeks after discontinuation of treatment, so a further course should not be considered until this time has elapsed. Patients are able to have longer courses of treatment (up to 24 weeks) or a repeat course as necessary, but it has been shown that no substantial additional benefit is expected beyond a cumulative treatment dose of 120–150 mg/kg.

What if my patient has a flare of their acne when starting isotretinoin?

All patients should be warned that this may happen in the first few weeks of their treatment. In very severe acne, this can be minimized by starting on a half dose (0.5 mg/kg/day), or by the use of topical or oral corticosteroids to manage a severe flare, should it occur.

What if my patient is slow to respond, or fails to respond to isotretinoin?

Check if your patient is taking the tablets! If so, ensure that the patient is on the full dose according to weight. Some patients will be slower to respond, and a prolonged course (up to 24 weeks) can be given, provided side effects are tolerable. Note that acne cysts and large nodules will often require physical treatments to improve their appearance.

ROSACEA

This is a disorder characterized by frequent flushing, persistent erythema and telangiectasia, with episodes of inflammation, papules and pustules, but *no comedones*.

Epidemiology

Rosacea is very common, affecting 10% of the population. It is mainly seen in fair-skinned individuals who easily blush, or have a 'high colour'. It is more common in women in their third and fourth decades.

Aetiology and pathogenesis

This is unclear, and probably due to many factors with the most likely being a vascular abnormality.

- Vascular abnormality — this has been proposed as possible vascular hyper-reactivity, or long-standing vascular damage from solar radiation.
- *Demodex* mite — the *Demodex* mite is present on everyone, but some studies have found higher concentrations on the skin of patients with rosacea. Treatment directed at the mite has, in some cases, led to clinical improvement, especially in HIV infected patients. However, it may be that a separate entity, *Demodex* folliculitis, has clinically resembled rosacea in HIV infection, thus confusing the clinical outcomes.
- *Helicobacter pylori* — it has been noticed that many patients treated with *H. pylori* eradication for peptic ulcer have co-incidental improvement in their rosacea. The role of *H. pylori* in rosacea is still unproven.

Clinical features (Figure 4.10)

The cheeks, nose, forehead and chin are most commonly affected, with occasional spread to scalp and torso.

It often progresses in a stepwise fashion:

- Transient erythema.
- Persistent erythema and telangiectasia.
- Papules and pustules.
- Chronic thickening and induration of skin.
- Rhinophyma.

Ocular rosacea

In ocular rosacea there may be irritation and redness of the conjunctiva, blepharitis, styes and, occasionally, keratitis. First line treatment is usually with artificial tears and systemic tetracyclines (Table 4.5).

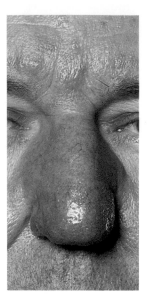

Figure 4.10
Rosacea. Note the erythematous papules and telangiectasia on the forehead, and rhinophyma on the nose.

Rhinophyma

Rhinophyma describes distortion of normal skin surface of the nose, which can lead to great cosmetic disfigurement. Once the active rosacea has been treated, surgical remodelling, with electrosurgery, CO_2 or Nd:Yag laser can be performed.

Differential diagnosis

- Acne vulgaris — comedones are also present.
- Systemic/discoid lupus erythematosus — no pustules occur. Scarring, scaling and follicular plugging are the prominent features of discoid lupus.
- Seborrhoeic dermatitis — the major feature is scaling, which occurs on the scalp, eyebrows and external ear canals.

Management

The management of rosacea is summarized in Table 4.5. In particular, the cosmetic appearance of this condition, and its effect on the patient, should be considered when deciding on management options.

Variants of rosacea

Steroid-induced rosacea

Prolonged facial application of potent topical steroid can induce rosacea. The steroid needs to be withdrawn (often with intermediate potency steroid initially). Concomitant use of

Table 4.5: Management of rosacea

Therapy	Top tips
Sunscreen	Avoiding alcohol, spicy foods and hot drinks may also reduce flushing
Topical metronidazole	Can irritate the skin
Oral antibiotics: Tetracyclines Erythromycin	See Acne Table 4.4
Topical sulphur/ Ketoconazole/ Demodex eradication	All may have some benefit as second/third line therapy
Isotretinoin	See Acne Table 4.4 and main text for acne
Cosmetic treatments: Cosmetic camouflage Pulsed dye laser	Both treatments used to conceal or cosmetically treat erythema on face

topical or systemic antibiotics, or topical tacrolimus, reduces the likelihood of the condition flaring on stopping steroid creams.

Rosacea fulminans ('pyoderma faciale')

This is a very severe variant of rosacea, mainly of adult females, with marked erythema, pustules and oedema, which can lead to severe scarring. It has been linked with use of the oral contraceptive pill and pregnancy, suggesting a hormonal trigger. Patients require treatment with systemic corticosteroids and isotretinoin (see Acne section for further information).

Perioral dermatitis

Small papules and pustules appear around the mouth, sparing the lip margins. There is also a peri-ocular variant (peri-ocular dermatitis). It is exacerbated by topical steroid use. Management consists of stopping any topical steroids (an initial flare may occur), and starting topical or systemic antibiotics, as one would in standard rosacea treatment (Table 4.5).

LICHENOID DISORDERS

Lichenoid describes the clinical appearance of a flat-topped, shiny, papular rash. It also describes the histological appearance of a band-like inflammatory infiltrate in the superficial dermis, with liquefaction of the basal layer. Its distinct histology usually makes a biopsy of such a rash helpful in its diagnosis. A lichenoid eruption can occur due to a number of causes (Box 4.6), and again histology can be helpful in distinguishing between the various causes. This section will discuss lichen planus only.

> **Box 4.6: Commoner causes of 'lichenoid' eruptions**
>
> - Lichen planus
> - Drug eruption — particularly gold, mepacrine, quinine, tetracyclines, thiazide diuretics, amlodipine
> - Graft versus host disease
> - Pityriasis lichenoides
> - Keratosis lichenoides chronica ('Nekam's disease')
> - Lichen nitidus
> - Lichen striatus
> - Mycosis fungoides (cutaneous T-cell lymphoma)

LICHEN PLANUS

Epidemiology

Seventy five percent of patients with cutaneous lichen planus have oral involvement, so *looking in the mouth is essential* and helpful in diagnosing the condition. Ten to twenty percent of patients develop oral lichen planus first, so often present to their dentist or the oral surgeons.

Pathogenesis

Lichen planus is a T-cell mediated autoimmune inflammatory condition. Its cause is unknown, although small studies have suggested a familial tendency, and also a possible association with hepatitis C. Oral lichen planus may be related to amalgam fillings.

Clinical features (Figure 4.11)

Shiny, flat-topped violaceous papules occur on the skin, in a variety of configurations. These can be small papules, linear or annular lesions. They are often itchy. Lichen planus can also display the Koebner phenomenon (Box 4.1). On the surface, a lace-like, white pattern is often seen — Wickham's striae. The papules can also become hyperpigmented, especially in darker skin types, and can become hypertrophic, particularly on the ankles and shins.

Differential diagnosis

A skin biopsy is very helpful in confirming a lichenoid eruption, and also in distinguishing its cause. Other conditions which should be considered are plane warts, lichenified eczema, lichen simplex chronicus, lupus erythematosus, psoriasis and secondary syphilis.

Lichen planus of mucous membranes

The mouth

In the mouth, lichen planus has the appearance of white lace-like patches, often symmetrically distributed. If the patient has co-existing lichen planus of the skin, it is

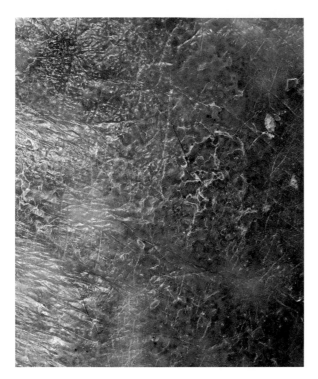

Figure 4.11
Lichen planus. A close up view showing the violaceous plaque topped by Wickham's striae.

reasonable to treat them in the first instance with topical corticosteroids to the mouth. A strong corticosteroid in a base designed for oral administration (e.g. triamcinolone in oral paste) is usually helpful. A patient with non-responding, atypical or asymmetrical lesions, particularly if they are a smoker, should be referred to the oral surgeons for consideration of biopsy. Remember that squamous cell carcinoma can occasionally arise in these lesions, so again atypical ulceration or new lumps in the mouth should be investigated.

Genital area

This can affect both sexes, but is more common on the vulva, and can be difficult to treat. At worst, the lesions on the vulva can ulcerate, causing painful scarring. A biopsy should be taken to differentiate it from lichen sclerosis, which can have a similar appearance.

Other sites

- Nails: In 10% of cases there is nail involvement, particularly of the finger nails, with ridging and thinning of the nail plate. The nail can be completely lost, or can form a 'pterygium' (severe narrowing of the nail resulting from partial destruction).
- Scalp: Lichen planus of the scalp can cause scarring alopecia and skin atrophy, and should be looked for (again a biopsy is very helpful) and managed early to try to avoid such permanent scarring.

71

Treatment of lichen planus

The first line treatment of localized areas of lichen planus is topical steroids, which can be occluded to increase potency and also to reduce rubbing of the affected area. Use of potent corticosteroids, especially under occlusion, carries the risk of skin atrophy, and topical immunosuppressants may be a useful alternative. More widespread or non-responsive lesions require systemic treatment, with oral corticosteroids in the first instance (unless contraindicated), or with retinoids, ciclosporin or PUVA as second line therapy.

ERYTHRODERMA

Erythroderma is defined as more than 90% involvement of the body surface by an inflammatory skin disease (Figure 4.12). It can occur, for example, in patients with chronic

Figure 4.12
Erythroderma.

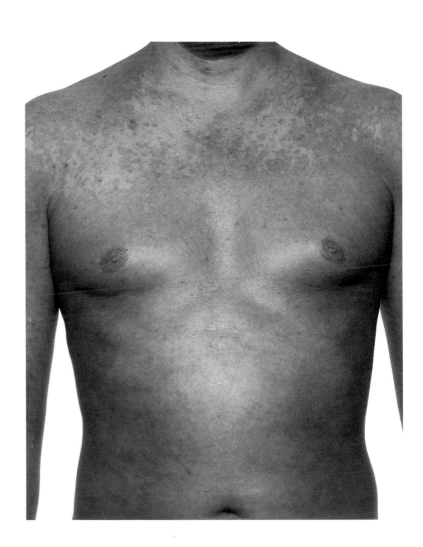

plaque psoriasis, who experience a trigger (e.g. infection/stress/withdrawal of topical or systemic corticosteroids or immunosuppressants). However, there are a number of other causes, summarized in Table 4.6.

It is important that the underlying cause is identified although in 8% of cases it is not found. Questions to ask in the history include previous and family history of skin disease, drug history (including over-the-counter medications) and systemic symptoms. General examination of the patient is essential (including lymph nodes) and a skin biopsy can be helpful if the cause is not obvious.

Management

Erythroderma is a *dermatological emergency*. The skin function has failed, and management is mainly supportive. The most important complications are:

- Loss of body heat — keep the patient warm. Try to get the patient nursed in a single cubicle as it is easier to keep the ambient temperature higher.
- Dehydration — plentiful oral fluids should be encouraged. Intravenous fluids should be considered if the patient is not drinking enough or is pyrexial. Liberal use of emollients is essential.
- Infection — weeping skin should be swabbed and treated with oral antibiotics. If the patient becomes pyrexial, a full septic screen should be performed (blood cultures/urine culture/throat swab/other depending on symptoms), but remember that just having the erythroderma can cause a pyrexia too.
- Loss of protein and increased energy requirements — increased nutrition, particularly protein supplements, should be given.
- Increased risk of deep vein thrombosis — if the patient is dehydrated and immobile, deep vein thrombosis prophylaxis should be considered.
- Find and treat underlying cause — this may involve stopping the offending drug, or starting immunosuppressive drugs, depending on the underlying condition.

Table 4.6: Commonest causes of erythroderma

	% of overall prevalence
Eczema (any type)	40
Psoriasis	25
Lymphoma and leukaemias	15
Drug reactions — particularly allopurinol, anticonvulsants, gold, penicillin, sulphonamides	10
Idiopathic	8
Pityriasis rubra pilaris/paraneoplastic (often late stage)/pemphigus foliaceous/ congenital ichthyoses	< 1

STEVENS–JOHNSON SYNDROME AND TOXIC EPIDERMAL NECROLYSIS

These are the more severe end of the 'erythema multiforme' spectrum, and are the most serious of *dermatological emergencies*. Patients usually present with macular, papular or urticarial lesions on the skin, sometimes with erosions affecting the mucous membranes. As you go further down the list (Box 4.7), the conditions become more severe, with more widespread skin erosions and skin loss, and more severe involvement of the mucous membranes. The mortality rate also increases, to a level of about 30–40% in toxic epidermal necrolysis (TEN). Stevens–Johnson syndrome (SJS) and TEN are usually due to drug reactions, and are often considered separately.

The most common drugs which can cause SJS or TEN are summarized in Box 4.8. There is an overlap between drugs which cause SJS and those which cause TEN, indeed SJS can evolve into TEN (so these patients should be monitored carefully).

Clinical features (Figure 4.13)

The patient is usually systemically unwell, often with a prodrome of fever, malaise and arthralgia. The most striking feature will be erosions of the lips and the inside of the

---

Box 4.7: *Spectrum of erythema multiforme*

Erythema multiforme	Mild
Stevens–Johnson syndrome (SJS)	↓
Toxic epidermal necrolysis (TEN)	Severe

Box 4.8

Commonest drugs which can cause Stevens–Johnson syndrome

- Sulphonamides
- Tetracyclines
- Penicillin
- Malaria prophylaxis drugs

Commonest drugs which can cause toxic epidermal necrolysis

- Sulphonamides
- NSAIDs
- Allopurinol
- Anticonvulsants
  - Barbiturates
  - Phenytoin
  - Carbamazepine
  - Lamotrigine
- Antiretroviral drugs
  - Nevirapine

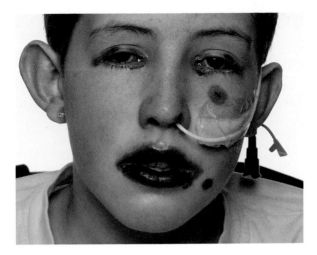

Figure 4.13
Stevens–Johnson syndrome. Note the conjunctival and oral erosions, and a typical erythema multiforme-like 'target lesion' on the left of the mouth.

mouth. The conjunctiva and genital areas can also be severely affected, so the patient should be specifically asked about symptoms in these areas.

As the skin begins to blister, it is useful to test it with 'Nikolsky's sign'. A positive result describes firm sliding pressure with a finger, which then separates normal-looking epidermis from the dermis producing an erosion. The presence of Nikolsky's sign indicates weakness and loss of cohesion within the epidermis at the dermo-epidermal junction. Nikolsky's sign is useful to assess any blistering condition, including the immunobullous diseases. A positive result indicates that the patient is more at risk of complications.

The most important steps would be:

- *Seek senior help*.
- Stop the offending drug.
- Supportive care of the patient's skin — this is the same as in the Erythroderma section. Correct fluid balance is of the utmost importance for these patients.
- Correct placement — patients with TEN should be managed in an intensive care setting, preferably in a burns unit.
- Care of mucous membranes — this may involve the patient being nil by mouth, requiring catheterization, or needing referral to ophthalmology.
- An excellent review is recommended by Chave et al.[13]

References

1. van de Kerkof PCM. The psoriasis area and severity index and alternative approaches for the assessment of severity. Br J Dermatol 1997; 137:661–663.
2. Lewis VJ, Finlay AY. Two decades experience of the psoriasis disability index (PDI). Dermatology 2005; 210:261–268.
3. Lewis VJ, Finlay AY. 10 years experience of the Dermatology Life Quality Index. JID Symp Proc 2004; 9:169–180.
4. Dermatology Life Quality Index. Online. Available: http://www.dermatology.org.uk

5. Psoriasis Association: Online. Available: http://www.psoriasis-association.org.uk

6. Williams HC, Burnley PGJ, Strachan D, Hay RJ. The UK working party's diagnostic criteria for atopic dermatitis. III. Independent hospital validation. Br J Dermatol 1994; 131:406–416.

7. Hanifin JM, Thurston M, Omoto M, et al. The eczema area and severity index (EASI): assessment of reliability in atopic dermatitis. Exper Dermatol 2001; 10:11–18.

8. Severity scoring of atopic dermatitis: the SCORAD index. Consensus report of the European Task Force on Atopic Dermatitis. Dermatol 1993; 186:23–31.

9. Lewis-Jones MS, Finlay AY. The Children's Dermatology Life Quality Index (CDLQI): Initial validation and practical use. Br J Dermatol 1995; 132:942–949.

10. National Eczema Society. Online. Available: http://www.eczema.org

11. Burke BM, Cunliffe WJ. The assessment of acne vulgaris – the Leeds technique. Br J Dermatol 1984; 111:83–92.

12. British Association of Dermatologists. Online. Available: http://www.bad.org.uk/healthcare/guidelines/

13. Chave TA, Mortimer NJ, Sladden MJ, Hall AP, Hutchinson PE. Toxic epidermal necrolysis: current evidence, practical management and future directions. Br J Dermatol 2005; 153:241–253.

Further reading

Bolognia JL, Jorizzo JL, Rapini RP, eds. Dermatology. London: Mosby; 2003.

Burns T, Breathnach S, Cox N, Griffiths C, eds. Rook's textbook of dermatology. 7th edn. Oxford: Blackwell Scientific; 2004.

Lebwohl M, Heymann WR, Berth-Jones J, Coulson I. Treatment of skin disease. 2nd edn. Edinburgh: Mosby; 2006.

Website

http://www.bad.org.uk/public/leaflets/

Paediatric dermatology

Sharon L. W. Blackford

INTRODUCTION

Children under the age of 16 make up 5–8% of referrals to a typical dermatology department in a UK district general hospital. While all trainees in dermatology will have had experience in adult medicine most will have had no paediatric training since they qualified as doctors. This can lead to a lack of confidence in dealing with children and with small infants especially. While textbooks, journals and courses can improve your knowledge of paediatric dermatology there is no substitute for hands on experience in a dedicated clinic to achieve a more confident approach to children.

The most common referral encountered in the paediatric dermatology clinic is a child with atopic eczema. This can vary from a small infant, in which case the diagnosis raises many questions and anxieties for the parents, to an older child or adolescent who may be very disgruntled to find they have not 'grown out' of their eczema as they had been promised. There are too many other dermatological conditions that can present in the paediatric population to be covered in this limited space, and there are several excellent textbooks that already do this very well (see Further reading). Instead this chapter will attempt to cover some of the aspects of paediatric dermatology which differ from general adult dermatology, and which all specialist registrars would be expected to cover during their attachment in a paediatric dermatology clinic.

HISTORY TAKING

When interviewing a child with a skin problem it is best not to make assumptions at the start of the consultation. First introduce yourself, then politely ask the adults with the child what their relationship to the patient is, as it could be a grandparent, older sibling or a child minder who brings the child to clinic. Find out by what name the child is usually known and use it when talking to the child and the family. Usually the mother brings the child and she gives the history. Older children may be able to contribute and should be encouraged to do so but younger children will soon get bored; there should be plenty of toys available for them to play with while the adults talk. This is useful to observe, as it will guide your examination of the child later. If the child is confident to leave their parents to play on the floor then they will probably let you examine them even if you have to get down to the floor to do so. However, if the child remains clinging to mum's leg, you are unlikely to get much co-operation by prising them away, and it is better to limit the examination to what you can see while they sit on the parent's knee.

History taking in children differs slightly from that for adults. There are some specific questions that need to be covered:

- Birth history: Was the pregnancy, labour and delivery normal?
- Birth weight.
- Feeding: Bottle or breast? Has weaning started? Has the diet been manipulated in any way? (e.g. change of formula milk, exclusion of cows' milk).
- Immunizations.
- Hospitalizations.
- Development: For older children which school do they attend? How are they getting on in school? For children under school age ask if the parents have any concerns about the child's development.
- Family history: A brief enquiry into other family members' health can be very valuable, e.g. other family members with an itchy rash suggests scabies, and knowing that a relative died of melanoma helps to explain why a simple naevus is causing so much anxiety. If an inherited disorder is suspected a more detailed family history should be taken (see Genetics and genetic counselling).

EXAMINATION (Figure 5.1)

Infants up to 18 months old are quite easy to examine on a couch or on mother's knee. Smiling and talking to the baby in a calm and friendly voice while you examine them will help even if they do not understand what you are saying. Toddlers, however, are a different matter! The 'terrible twos' are so called for a reason. At this age children are starting to learn some independence but this also brings with it fears of insecurity. This conflict can result in clingy behaviour, to a person or to an object, e.g. a security blanket or toy. Toddlers may also display their independence by temper tantrums and refusal to co-operate with your attempts to examine them. Get down to their level on the floor, and engage the child in play to distract them and gain their trust first. If they still refuse to let you see their 'bad skin', it may be best to defer examination to another occasion. It is not usually necessary to strip a child completely, it is often better to examine the skin a little at a time starting with hands and arms to build up their trust. You may not be able to carry out the examination in any set order, you may start with hands and arms and then the child will show you their feet; be prepared to alter your normal examination technique as required.

Over the age of 3, most children will respond well to smiles and discussion about their favourite toy, football team or pop star depending on their age. However, in adolescents it can sometimes feel like dealing with a toddler again. Try to bear in mind that the sullen young person in a baseball hat who can only communicate in grunts may actually be withdrawn and depressed about his or her skin complaint.

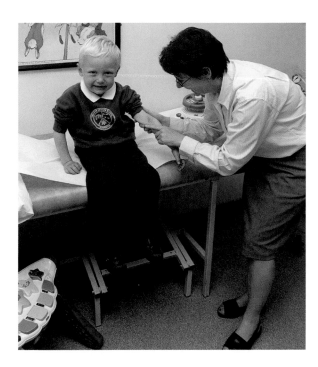

Figure 5.1
Examination of a toddler.

THE ROLE OF THE CLINICAL NURSE SPECIALIST

During the last 10–15 years, one of the major changes to dermatology practice in the UK has been the development of the role of dermatology specialist nurses. In paediatric dermatology especially, the clinical nurse specialist (CNS) can play a vital role in patient and parent education, particularly for children with atopic eczema. Often, the reason for referral is poor compliance with treatment; this is nearly always because the parents have had inadequate information or guidance on how to use the treatments. In addition to educational advice about eczema and the treatment regimen required, the CNS can also provide follow-up support in person and via the telephone, thus freeing up the doctors to do what they do best.

Trainees should take the opportunity to spend time with the CNS, to observe practical demonstrations of emollients and wet wrapping for example. Parents and children like to try out different emollients in the clinic, and they may leave the nurse consultation with several samples to try at home, thus encouraging better compliance (Figure 5.2).

GROWTH MONITORING

All children attending hospital should be weighed and measured as a routine; the paediatric dermatology clinic is no exception (Figure 5.3). The appropriate weight and height charts, which are gender and age specific, should be available in the clinic and are used to plot

Figure 5.2
The clinical nurse specialist has a particular role in patient and/or parent education.

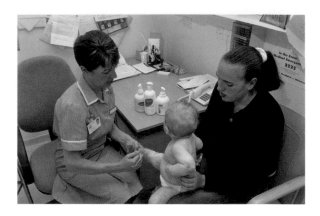

Figure 5.3
Measuring height and weight should be routine in the paediatric clinic.

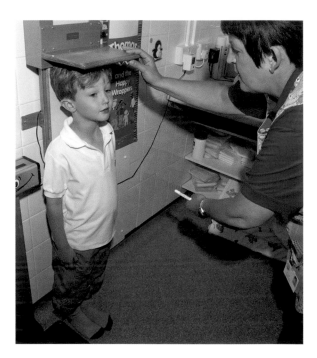

growth over time. For any child using potent topical steroids or on systemic medication careful monitoring of growth while on treatment is mandatory. Growth monitoring is also important when any form of dietary restriction is being used (Figure 5.4).

Excessive height is usually familial, but a tall girl referred with early onset acne may have precocious puberty or isolated adrenarche, thus measuring the child could prompt referral for endocrine investigations.

Obesity in childhood is now becoming increasingly common, and Type 2 diabetes mellitus is being seen in teenagers and younger children. Insulin resistance is associated with many skin abnormalities so the child's first point of referral to secondary care could be the dermatology clinic.

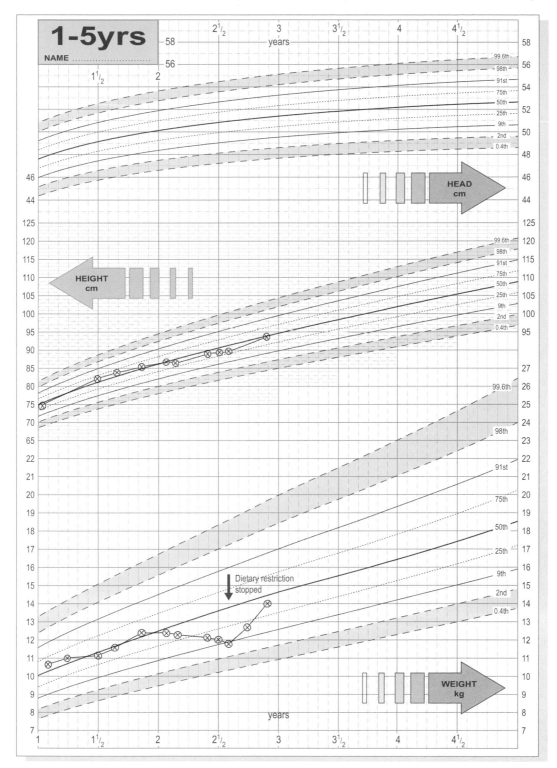

Figure 5.4
A growth chart is shown of a 2 year old with atopic eczema. He had been on a severely restricted diet of fruit, vegetables and 'rice milk' on the advice of a complementary therapist. His weight had fallen from the 50th percentile to around the 9th percentile. His eczema responded to conventional topical treatment and he gained weight when he was back on a normal diet. © Child Growth Foundation.

DIETARY ADVICE AND MONITORING

Many parents will ask about the role of diet in controlling their child's skin as it is a commonly held belief that food allergy causes most skin complaints! In the vast majority of skin diseases this is not the case, but referral to a dietician is helpful in a number of conditions, and vital in several others. These include gluten sensitivity which can present as dermatitis herpetiformis, children with dystrophic epidermolysis bullosa which involves the oral mucosa, and children with actual food allergy. However, the most frequent reason for referral to the paediatric dietetic service is for a child with atopic eczema (Box 5.1).

Diet in atopic eczema

It is a popular misconception that atopic eczema is caused by food allergy and many parents will attend the paediatric dermatology clinic hoping that allergy tests will reveal the cure for their child's eczema. In reality, the role of food hypersensitivity is much more controversial and complicated. While food allergy is never the cause of atopic eczema, hypersensitivity to one or more foods is one of the triggers that can cause a flare-up of eczema (Table 5.1).

Many parents will have already tried some form of dietary manipulation before being seen, often stopping cows' milk, but not always removing all sources of cows' milk protein or carrying on for sufficient time. Soya milk is often used as a milk substitute, and may have been suggested by the health visitor or GP. However, allergy to soya can occur in 10% of children with cows' milk allergy.

Allergy testing with skin prick tests and RAST tests is also notoriously unhelpful. False positives are common in active eczema, and false negatives can occur, as not all food intolerance is IgE mediated.

Box 5.1: When to try a diet in atopic eczema

- Child under 2 years old (especially infants still exclusively breast fed).
- Parents very keen to try diet.
- Widespread eczema.
- History of food intolerance.

Table 5.1: Which foods are most likely to cause reactions in atopic eczema?

Low risk (common weaning foods)	→	Medium risk	→	High risk (severe reactions can occur)
Baby rice	Cereals, rusks	Citrus fruits	Cows' milk	Peanuts
Vegetables	Meat, fish	Strawberries	Goats' milk	Shellfish
Apple, pear		Tomatoes	Eggs	Kiwi fruit

One practical approach to diet is to try a limited exclusion diet, often cows' milk and egg, for a defined period of 6 to 8 weeks. At the end of this trial the excluded foods are reintroduced one at a time and the child can be monitored to observe whether the eczema improves with exclusion and then flares as the foods are reintroduced. The advice and support of a paediatric dietician is vital, first by educating the parents and suggesting an appropriate milk substitute, and in ensuring the child is having the appropriate intake of protein, calcium and other nutrients.

GENETICS AND GENETIC COUNSELLING

The field of genetics has seen a revolution in the last two decades, and continues to grow rapidly. In recent years the genetic basis of many inherited skin conditions has been identified. Many of these genodermatoses are rare. An individual dermatologist may only see the condition once in their career, and therapeutic options are often very limited. The families affected by these conditions, however, may benefit from the advances in genetic testing, for example by getting a definitive diagnosis, by receiving genetic counselling, and prenatal testing. As we understand more about the molecular basis of these conditions, the more likely it is that new treatments will be discovered.

When seeing a child with a skin condition that could be inherited, the first step is to take and record a detailed family history.

Here are some examples:

- Naevoid basal cell carcinoma syndrome (Gorlin syndrome, Gorlin–Goltz syndrome) (Figure 5.5a). An autosomal dominant condition. The PTCH gene, a tumour suppressor gene, located on chromosome 9q22.3-q31 is the site of the mutation. This results in numerous basal cell carcinomas at a young age. Other features include jaw cysts (first seen around puberty), palmar and plantar pits and skeletal abnormalities. Medulloblastoma occurs in 5% of infants with naevoid basal cell carcinoma syndrome. Prenatal and pre-symptomatic diagnosis is possible by gene tracking, depending on DNA availability from other family members.
- Xeroderma pigmentosum (Figure 5.5b). An autosomal recessive condition. There are seven different complementation groups (A to G) and XP variant, all with variable mutations at different chromosomal locations. Diagnosis is made by demonstrating abnormal DNA repair after ultra violet radiation of cultured fibroblasts. The clinical picture is a child with photosensitivity, early onset of skin cancers, pigmentary changes with marked freckling, and conjunctivitis. Ataxia, deafness and mental decline occur in complementation group A and are progressive. It is a rare condition, more common if the parents are consanguinous. Prenatal testing is possible.
- X-linked ichthyosis (steroid sulphatase deficiency) (Figure 5.5c). An X-linked recessive disorder, so the condition is seen in males. Carrier females are unaffected or may have corneal opacities and mild skin changes. Brown scaly skin occurs and is most noticeable in the flexures from approximately 6 months of age (Figure 5.6). The faulty gene on the X chromosome codes for the enzyme steroid sulphatase. Lack of the enzyme leads to

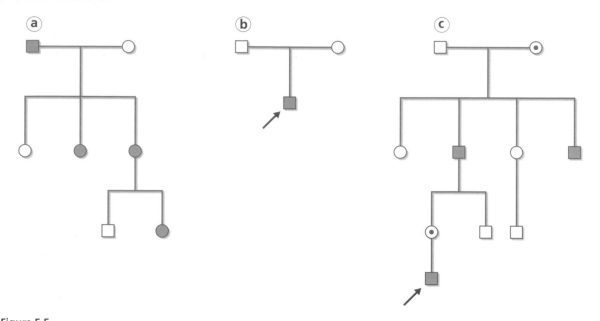

Figure 5.5
(a) Family tree demonstrating three generations affected in naevoid basal cell carcinoma syndrome. (b) Family tree of patient with xeroderma pigmentosum. (c) Family tree in X-linked ichthyosis.

Figure 5.6
Typical brown scales in flexures in X-linked ichthyosis.

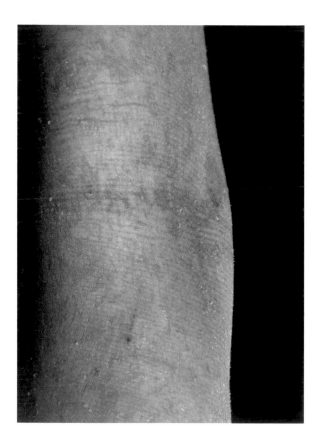

accumulation of cholesterol sulfate and high plasma levels are diagnostic. Low enzyme activity in the placenta leads to low levels of oestriol in maternal plasma and urine, with possible slow progression of labour when an affected male is being born.

PRESCRIBING FOR CHILDREN

Many of the topical and systemic drugs used to treat dermatology patients have not been specifically tested for paediatric use and many are unlicensed for use in children, particularly under 2 years of age. The diseases they are used for may be different in children and the formulations may have to be altered, for example tablets may have to be crushed. Nevertheless these drugs are often used, but some special considerations have to be taken into account when prescribing for children. The British National Formulary for Children should be used as a reference guide.

The epidermis in a full-term infant is well developed and has excellent barrier properties, but in a pre-term infant the stratum corneum is poorly developed, especially in those born before 24 weeks of gestation. This results in an increased rate of transepidermal water loss (TEWL), which causes problems with fluid regulation, temperature control and increased absorption of topical therapies. Babies and young children also have an increased body surface to weight ratio compared to adults; this means they are more likely to suffer systemic side effects from topically applied drugs. Apart from skin maturity, the other important factors that affect drug penetration are listed (Box 5.2).

Some drugs known to cause toxicity in children after topical application:

- Adrenaline (epinephrine): Local application to a bleeding circumcision site in a 2-day-old boy resulted in local pallor and tachycardia.
- Corticosteroids: Side effects are well documented and widely known about by the general public. As a result 'steroid phobia' is common and leads to much under-use. Side effects are more likely if potent or super potent steroids are used, and if applied for prolonged periods and/or under occlusion.
    - Local:
        - Striae and atrophy of skin
        - Infection
        - Hirsutism and acne
        - Hypopigmentation
        - Rebound flare of inflammation after discontinuation.
    - Systemic: (very rarely seen)
        - Cushing's syndrome
        - Hypothalamic-pituitary axis suppression
        - Glaucoma and cataracts
        - Failure to thrive.
- Immunomodulators: Tacrolimus ointment 0.1% (adults) and 0.03% (children); pimecrolimus 1% cream — both are licensed from age 2 years for short-term use in eczema. A tingling or burning sensation is quite common on initial use but often

> **Box 5.2:** *Factors influencing drug permeability through skin*
>
> ■ Age
> ■ Site: eyelid > forearm > sole of foot: flexures greater than other sites
> ■ Damage to skin: lichenification reduces permeation: inflammation increases permeation
> ■ Drug type: pH, particle size, water or lipid solubility
> ■ Vehicle type: ointment, cream, gel or lotion
> ■ Application method: occlusion under plastic increases topical steroid absorption ×10–100 times

improves. Local infections may be more likely, but the main concern of many clinicians is whether long-term use could increase the risk of skin malignancy. UV light avoidance is recommended.

- Iodine: Widely used as an antiseptic. When used in neonates or over large areas of denuded skin (e.g. burns) can cause abnormal thyroid function.
- Neomycin: Antibiotic well known to be ototoxic when given systemically, but there have been reports of deafness after topical treatment too.
- Salicylic acid: Preparations of salicylic acid are used as keratolytics in a wide range of skin complaints. They can cause salicylism in children, especially if applied over a large area of skin in a young child. Salicylate poisoning is more commonly due to accidental aspirin ingestion. In a child salicylism is potentially more serious than in an adult as metabolic acidosis is more likely.
- Scabicides: Lindane can cause CNS toxicity in infants and there are reports of aplastic anaemia following its use. It is less effective than permethrin 5% cream, which is the treatment of choice for children with scabies in the UK and is well tolerated. Malathion has also been reported to cause toxicity and hyperglycaemia in children but this was when applied as a 50% solution; the 0.5% liquid usually causes few problems.
- Topical anaesthetics: EMLA (Eutectic Mixture of Local Anaesthetics) contains 2.5% lidocaine (lignocaine) and 2.5% prilocaine and is widely used prior to venepuncture, prior to injection of anaesthetic for skin surgery and before laser treatment of skin in children. It requires application under occlusion for 1 to 5 hours to be effective. Local effects include erythema and dermatitis; systemically it has been associated with methaemoglobinaemia in infants under 3 months of age. Benzocaine gel can cause methaemoglobinaemia after application to skin or mucous membranes. Infants are more commonly affected.

COMMUNICATION WITH OTHER PROFESSIONALS

Children can be referred to the paediatric dermatology clinic by a number of routes. The most common is a referral direct from the child's general practitioner (GP) or practice nurse, but health visitors, paediatricians, accident and emergency doctors amongst others can ask for a dermatology opinion. A letter detailing the consultation should always be sent on to the GP as well as to the person who referred the child, preferably within 2 working days.

Some dermatologists also send a copy to the family and this can be very helpful as a reminder for the parents especially if many different topics of discussion took place.

For example, on a first visit, when seeing a child suffering from atopic eczema it is quite routine to cover the following topics with the family:

Avoidance of irritants.
Use of emollients.
Use of topical steroids of different strengths at different sites.
Role of allergen avoidance.
The role of diet.
Risk of asthma developing.
Prognosis.

Other professionals likely to be involved with the child should also be informed; in pre-school children this is often the health visitor. The community paediatrician or schools medical officer can be sent copies of correspondence once the child is attending school. This is valuable if the child's condition limits their activity in school in some way or dictates that a different uniform is worn by the child, e.g. photosensitive conditions, blistering disorders. If treatment in the school day is required, extra training for school personnel or extra help may be required, as teachers will not apply creams or administer medicines to children. There may be a school nurse in large secondary schools to supervise older children applying or taking their own medication but in most primary schools they may not feel they are equipped to deal with these problems. If the parents give their consent, a letter to the head teacher outlining the issues can be very helpful; send a copy to the school's medical officer.

CHILD ABUSE

Good communication with other agencies and professional colleagues is particularly important when any form of child abuse is suspected (Box 5.3). Skin signs in physical abuse include bruising, scalds, cigarette burns and welts. Whilst it is common for infants when they start walking around the age of 12 months to have bruising on the legs and head, it is unusual to get bruises on the arms or chest. Gripping and shaking a baby produces fingertip bruises on the chest or arms. If non-accidental injury is suspected the child should be admitted immediately to a place of safety, usually hospital. There is no

---

Box 5.3: Types of child abuse

- Physical abuse
- Child sexual abuse
- Neglect
- Emotional abuse
- Munchausen syndrome by proxy

need to confront the parents with your suspicions at this stage, and most parents will agree to the child's admission to hospital. Further investigations to rule out other causes such as bleeding disorders can be made and enquiries by the child protection team can be carried out. It is very important that accurate and full documentation of any injuries and explanations given by the parents for those injuries are made. Encourage the child to talk, but do not ask leading questions or prompt them. If the child discloses to you that they are being abused do not promise to keep this a secret.

Other features which should raise suspicions of child abuse include:

• Delay in seeking medical care.
• History vague or keeps changing.
• History not consistent with child's injuries.
• Parental unconcern with child's injuries or hostility to further investigation.
• Injuries of different ages.

Risk factors for abuse are given in Box 5.4. Although abuse is more commonly reported in lower socioeconomic groups it can occur in all social classes. The mean age for an abused child is 6 years old, but under the age of 2 years abuse is more likely to lead to serious injury or death. All NHS trusts in the UK will have a child protection policy and procedures document, which should be available and will detail local arrangements for referrals to social services.

Even if a child is not in immediate danger, you might see a child who is dirty or unkempt, causing you to have concerns about neglect. You could have seen them because of head louse infestation and secondary infection, or nappy rash due to poor hygiene for example. You should talk to your consultant first; if this is not possible speak to the GP or the health visitor by telephone. They can visit the family at home to assess the situation and if necessary involve the community paediatric and/or social services. In some circumstances social services are involved with the family already and liaison with the social work team is very helpful; the social worker may accompany the family to the hospital to ensure they attend for example.

On the other hand, a dermatology opinion may be sought in cases of suspected abuse, when in fact there is another explanation for the skin signs. In the past, cases of vulval lichen sclerosus have been assumed by non-dermatologists to be due to sexual abuse. Other cases include bullous impetigo mistaken for cigarette burns, Mongolian blue spot thought

Box 5.4: *Risk factors for child abuse*

■ Parents suffered deprivation or abuse as children
■ Teenage pregnancy
■ Unwanted pregnancy
■ Premature birth or illness/disability
■ Lack of family or friends to give support
■ Drug and alcohol misuse
■ Poverty

to be due to bruising and striae or stretch marks across the back of a teenage boy thought to be due to beatings with a stick by his physical education teacher.

Further reading

British National Formulary for Children. London: British Medical Association, Royal Pharmaceutical Society of Great Britain, Royal College of Pediatricians and Child Health and the Neonatal and Paediatric Pharmacists Group; 2005. Online. Available: www.bnfc.org

Bruckner AL, Frieden IJ. Haemangiomas of infancy. J Am Acad Dermatol 2003; 48:477–493.

Harper J, Oranje A, Prose N, eds. Textbook of pediatric dermatology. 2nd edn. Oxford: Blackwell Science; 2006.

Higgins E, du Vivier A. Skin disease in childhood and adolescence. Oxford: Blackwell Science; 1996.

Hull D, Johnston DI. Essential paediatrics. 4th edn. Edinburgh: Churchill Livingstone; 1999.

Neonatal and Paediatric Pharmacists Group. Medicines for children. London: Royal College of Paediatrics and Child Health Publication; 2003.

Noren P. Habit reversal: a turning point in the treatment of atopic dermatitis. Clin Exp Dermatol 1995; 20:2–5.

Contact dermatitis

Nicolas G. Nicolaou and Mahbub M. U. Chowdhury

6

INTRODUCTION

Exposure of skin to external agents can cause many morphologically different skin reactions. These include acne, urticaria, lichenoid eruptions, hyper- or hypopigmentation but also dermatitis or eczema.

The dermatitis seen after contact with an external agent can be either irritant or allergic in nature. An example of irritant dermatitis would be exposure of skin to acids. The direct reaction is due to direct damage to the skin rather than an allergy. In an allergic reaction the skin is sensitized to an agent, for example nickel, and subsequent exposure to this agent tends to cause allergic contact dermatitis.

The mechanism of the reaction is different in allergic contact dermatitis (ACD) and irritant contact dermatitis (ICD). ACD is a type 4 or delayed hypersensitivity reaction while ICD is the result of localized toxic effects of an irritant on the skin. To complicate matters in chronic forms both ICD and ACD can look quite similar clinically, are difficult to differentiate and indeed may co-exist.

ICD accounts for approximately 80% of all contact dermatitis, while ACD accounts for the remaining 20%. This is often in contrast with what the patient may think, as they frequently suspect an allergy.

Allergy tests include prick testing (type 1 hypersensitivity reaction) and patch testing (for contact dermatitis and delayed hypersensitivity reaction).

PRICK TESTING

This test is primarily used to detect allergens involved in the occurrence of type 1 or acute hypersensitivity reactions. The classical example of this is contact urticarial reaction to an allergen such as nuts or latex. This test is also sometimes used in the investigation of asthma and hay fever for other allergens such as house dust mite. The antigen (allergen) binds to a specific IgE antibody on the surface of the dermal mast cells. This causes degranulation of the mast cells and release of histamine and other vasoactive substances leading to dermal oedema, known as a weal, surrounded by an erythematous flare.

Technique

In this test a small needle is used to gently prick the skin through a drop of fluid containing a known allergen. This lets a very small quantity of allergen into the dermis. It is usually carried out on the forearm, although with young children the back may be more suitable so they cannot see what is happening. The test is not painful and results are immediately available.

Solutions containing antigens are available commercially for a number of allergens including latex, mites, animal fur, moulds, trees, grasses, herbs and numerous food products.

In most cases, clinics have purified liquid forms of the allergen but sometimes, for example in the case of foods, the patient may be asked to bring in a fresh sample. Different foods can be brought into clinic in a refrigerator icecube box in separate compartments to prevent contamination.

Interpretation of prick tests

A positive reaction to the skin prick test occurs when the skin around the needle prick becomes pruritic and erythematous with the development of a weal (Figure 6.1a, b). The weal reaches its maximum size in about 15 to 20 minutes and the reaction fades within a few hours. The larger the weal, the more likely that the patient is allergic to the allergen. Also included in skin testing is a negative and positive control. The negative control is a saline (salt-water) solution, to which a response is not expected. If, however, a patient reacts to a negative control, then this will indicate that the skin is, for what ever reason, extremely sensitive and that the results need to be interpreted with the utmost care.

The positive control solution contains histamine, to which everyone is expected to react. A negative response to skin prick testing usually indicates that the patient is not sensitive to that allergen. Negative reactions may occur if the patient is taking antihistamines or medication that block the effect of histamine. Also the skin in some elderly people may not be capable of reacting. Patients will be asked to avoid taking any antihistamines a few days prior to the test.

For reasons not yet fully understood, skin prick testing with food allergens is less reliable than with some other allergens such as dust and pollens, in that false negative reactions can occur.

A blood test to look for specific IgE can also be used instead of a prick testing in the following cases:

- The patient has a risk of an anaphylactic (shock) reaction, so skin prick testing would be considered unsuitable.
- When extensive eczema makes skin prick testing impractical.

91

Figure 6.1
(a) Positive skin prick test to latex. (b) Close up view of positive reaction.

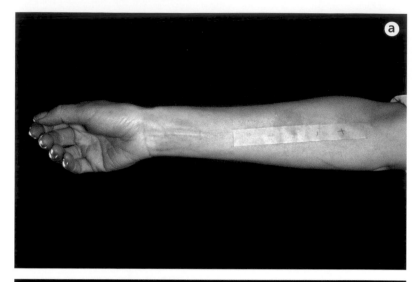

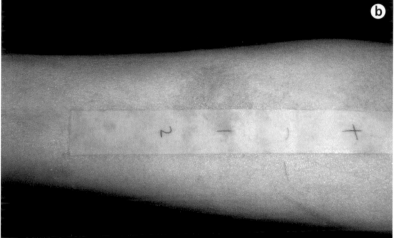

- When antihistamine medication cannot be stopped because of the severity of the symptoms.
- Where unusual and rare allergens are suspected.

A positive specific IgE test will help to confirm the allergy. Unfortunately a negative test cannot completely exclude an allergy and a prick test may also become necessary.

Key points for prick tests

- Used for testing type 1 hypersensitivity allergic reactions such as latex.
- Does not test for contact dermatitis.
- Allergen introduced intradermally.
- Positive if there is formation of weal.
- Resuscitation facilities must be available due to anaphylaxis risk.

PATCH TESTING

Jadassohn first described the technique of patch testing 100 years ago. Since then the technique has been constantly improved and further developed with many more allergens identified and tested. Patch testing is the gold standard for diagnosing ACD and the concept remains the same today. Allergens are applied to the skin, in a controlled fashion, in order to reproduce any possible allergic contact reaction and thus diagnosing ACD.

ACD can affect any age group and frequency of allergy to specific allergens can vary depending on previous or current exposure. Nickel allergy is commoner in women than men because of their greater exposure to jewellery. Similarly there is variability in different regions due to different habits and government legislation. Allergy to preservatives in cosmetics is such an example. The work environment plays an important role as workers can be exposed to different agents and can be sensitized. These occupational contact allergies can be quite specific and unique to these work groups.

As can be seen, there is no one series of allergens that could cover all possible allergens as these vary according to the country, occupation, hobbies and also with the area of the skin affected. Indications for patch testing are listed in Box 6.1.

It is important to take a good history and the clinician should ask questions about exposures at work and home including hobbies. A suggested history format is shown in Box 6.2.

Box 6.1: Indications for patch testing

- Atopic dermatitis
- Hand dermatitis
- Other dermatoses, e.g. discoid, stasis, seborrheoic
- Specific site dermatitis, e.g. eyelids, foot, perineal
- Occupational dermatitis

Box 6.2: Important history points in patch testing clinic

- Site of onset of dermatitis
- Duration and spread of dermatitis
- Relieving/exacerbating factors including holidays/work
- Past history: atopy, psoriasis, suspected nickel/perfume allergy
- Presence of vesicles/blisters
- Response to treatments
- Occupational details: potential allergen/irritant exposures; personal protection, e.g. gloves, overalls; handwashing frequency; barrier creams/soaps
- Hobbies (adults and children): potential exposures, e.g. oils, plants, gloves in sport

Technique

Patch testing aims to reproduce, in miniature, an eczematous eruption. The perfect patch test should give no false positives and no adverse reactions or sensitization to the allergens. The technique initially varied considerably in different centres.

The allergens are usually placed in Finn chambers (Figure 6.2). These are 8 mm aluminium pots, which provide good occlusion because of the chamber design. These chambers are placed on an adhesive tape and are available in strips of 10. Other similar preparations are also available.

The relevant allergens to be tested are then selected according to the history, occupation and location of the problem. Individual allergens can be bought commercially and these can then be placed in the chambers. A group of filled chamber strips constitutes a patch test series.

The concentration of the allergen chosen should be below the irritant concentration but above the allergic concentration. As the irritant threshold can vary in different populations, the strength used in the patch tests has been reached by trial and error over many years. Despite the best efforts to quantify the 'right' concentration, false positives and false negatives may still occur. This is inevitable as there is a range of thresholds within the normal population.

Once the patch test series to be tested are ready these can then be placed onto the skin. The most common site used is the upper back (Figure 6.3a, b). The patient should not be sunburned in this area or have applied topical corticosteroids for 1 week. Systemic corticosteroids and antihistamines should be avoided if possible during testing. Placement of the patch tests series requires some training. As they need to remain on the back for 2 days, the patches are placed on the back with the adhesive tape that the chambers are already 'stuck' to and then reinforced with more low irritant adhesive tape such as Scanpor. A diagram map of where the patch tests are placed is recorded for future reference.

Figure 6.2
Finn chamber allergens ready to be applied to back.

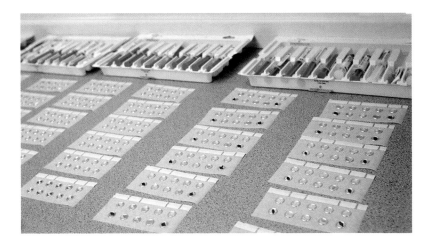

The patient is then asked to keep the back as dry as possible, avoiding excessive sweating and to keep the patches secure until the second visit after 2 days. When the patient returns 2 days later the patches are inspected to check if they have remained in place and whether there was adequate contact between the chambers and the back.

As the patches are removed their position is re-marked in order to identify the location of particular allergens, using a skin marker pen. Any positive reactions are scored according to the international grading system (Box 6.3). The patient is then asked to keep their back dry until the final reading which can be performed between 3 days and 2 weeks after initial application of the allergens. At the second reading, the map is used and any positive reactions are graded.

Positive reactions are caused by previous exposure at some time in the patient's life and may or may not be relevant to the current presenting problem of the patient. Some of the allergens are discussed later but it is important to remember that a patient may have contact with these at home, at work or at a recreational environment. Often the relevance is not clear at first and may require some detective work by the patient and doctor. Nevertheless the names and information sheets of the positive allergens should be given to

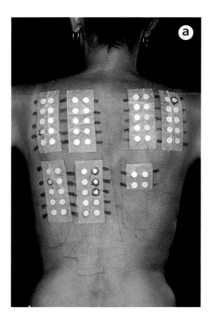
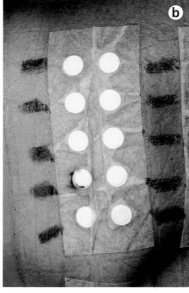

Figure 6.3
(a) Patches applied to patient's back. (b) One set of 10 allergens applied to back.

Box 6.3: Scheme for interpretation of patch testing results

– Negative reaction
? Doubtful reaction
+ Weak reaction (non-vesicular)
++ Strong reaction (oedematous or vesicular)
+++ Extreme reaction (ulcerative or bullous)
IR Irritant reaction
NT Not tested

the patient. These information sheets are also available online from the British Association of Dermatologists at www.bad.org.uk. The patient should try to avoid the positive allergens although 100% avoidance may be impossible.

In a perfect situation, only true positive and relevant reactions should occur and all allergens identified. Practically, however, recording and interpreting the results may be difficult as there may be false positive, marginal positive or irritant reactions. Moreover, an important allergen may have been missed in the patch testing as it was not identified from the initial clinical history.

In doubtful relevance, a repeated open application test (ROAT) is recommended. The test material can be applied to the skin of the antecubital space of the upper arm twice daily for a week. In most cases of contact allergy, an itchy papular dermatitis will develop.

PATCH TEST SERIES AND ALLERGENS

The International Contact Dermatitis Research Group was founded in 1967 and the main aim of the group was to provide a standardization of routine patch testing. A standard patch test series was put together in the 1960s in order to standardize patch testing. The aim of this series was to test an individual patient to the most common allergens encountered in the environment. Additional series can be added to the standard series if the investigator feels this is necessary.

There are three major standard series used around the world. The European standard series (25 allergens), the North American standard series (20 allergens) and the Japanese standard series (25 allergens). The standard series that is generally used in Europe is shown with brief details about the allergens (Table 6.1). In the United Kingdom, the British Contact Dermatitis Society (BCDS) standard series (39 allergens) is used (Box 6.4). Details are available on the BCDS website (www.bcds.org.uk).

Using a standard series has several advantages. Occasionally the patient omits an important part of the history which he or she can recall after the allergen is identified. Furthermore, if a patient is seen in another clinic the attending doctor will know what the tests were and therefore avoid miscommunication. Using a standard series allows comparative studies in different countries. The disadvantages include a possible downgrading of the importance of good history taking and possibly inducing sensitization to some of the additional allergens tested.

There are many patch test series available commercially. A list of available series is shown in Box 6.5. The allergens are available from several commercial companies which include TROLAB (www.hermal.de) and Chemotechnique (www.chemotechnique.se).

Interpreting patch tests results

This is usually the difficult part of the consultation and requires considerable skill and experience. Usually 4 days after the patch test series is put on the skin the final results are

Table 6.1

European standard battery	Main uses
Potassium dichromate	Tanning leather, cement
4-Phenylenediamine base	Azo dye intermediate, hair dye
Thiuram mix	Rubber accelerator, fungicides
Neomycin sulfate	Antibiotic in creams
Cobalt(II) chloride hexahydrate	Metal
Benzocaine	Local anaesthetic in creams
Nickelsulfate hexahydrate	Metal
Clioquinol	Synthetic anti-infective agent
Colophony	Pine resin, adhesives, printing ink
Paraben mix	Preservatives in creams
N-Isopropyl-N-phenyl-4-phenylenediamine (IPPD)	Black rubber chemical
Wool alcohols	Ointment base in creams
Mercapto mix	Rubber additives
Epoxy resin	Resin in adhesives, paint, insulation
Balsam of Peru	Fragrance and flavouring agent
4-tert-Butylphenolformaldehyde resin (PTBP)	Resin in adhesives
2-Mercaptobenzothiazole	Rubber chemical
Formaldehyde	Disinfectants, cosmetic preservatives
Fragrance mix	Fragrances
Sesquiterpene lactone mix	Plants
Quaternium 15	Formaldehyde releaser
Primin	Main allergen in primula dermatitis
5-Chloro-2-methyl-4-isothiazolin-3-one	Preservative in oils and creams
Budesonide	Non-halogenated steroid
Tixocortol-21-pivalate	Topical steroids (hydrocortisone)

read. The responses are seen and graded as positive (Figure 6.4a, b), negative or irritant (Box 6.3).

Doubtful or uncertain reactions may need to be repeated to check reproducibility, including serial dilution testing. Control testing may be necessary, and also open application tests can be useful. Pustular reactions usually indicate irritation and are not uncommon with metal allergens such as nickel and cobalt, occurring mainly in atopic patients.

To diagnose allergic contact dermatitis two significant steps should occur:

1. Identify a positive reaction to the patch test.
2. Demonstrate the clinical relevance.

Relevance can be determined through the process of reviewing exposures and products. Allergens may have past or current relevance. For example, a patient with a positive colophony patch test may have past relevance if he previously had a reaction to the adhesive of sticky plaster, but not current relevance if the current problem is unrelated. On the other hand, a positive colophony patch test may be of current relevance in a patient with a generalized eczematous eruption who had cut his pine hedge the weekend before this developed.

Box 6.4: British Contact Dermatitis Society standard series

■ Potassium dichromate	0.5%
■ Neomycin sulphate	20%
■ Thiuram mix	1%
■ p-Phenylenediamine	1%
■ Cobalt chloride	1%
■ Caine mix III	3.5%
■ Formaldehyde	1%
■ Rosin (Colophony)	20%
■ Quinolone mix	6%
■ Myroxylon Pereirae	25%
■ IPPD	0.1%
■ Wool alcohols	30%
■ Mercapto mix	2%
■ Epoxy resin	1%
■ Parabens mix	16%
■ PTBP resin	1%
■ Fragrance mix I	8%
■ Quaternium 15	1%
■ Nickel sulphate	5%
■ Me + Cl isothiazolinone	0.02% aqueous
■ Mercaptobenzothiazole	2%
■ Primin	0.01%
■ Sesquiterpene lactone mix	0.1%
■ Chlorocresol	1%
■ BromoNitropropaneDiol	0.25%
■ Cetearyl alcohol	5%
■ Fusidic acid	2%
■ Tixocortol-21-pivalate	0.1%
■ Budesonide	0.01%
■ Imidazolidinylurea	2%
■ Diazolidinylurea	2%
■ Methyldibromoglutaronitrile	0.3%
■ Ethylenediamine	1%
■ Chloroxylenol (PCMX)	0.5%
■ Carba mix	3%
■ Disperse Blue Mix 106/124	1%
■ Fragrance Mix II	14%
■ Lyral	5%
■ Compositae mix	2%

All dilutions in petrolatum unless stated.

It is worth keeping in mind that some allergens like gold may be late reactants and may come up after 4 days, so in some cases it might be worth arranging for a further reading the following week.

Similarly, relevance can be unknown in a patient with a reaction but no identifiable connection with the patient. It is worth considering the possibility of a false positive reaction as this can occur and is not infrequent. Mixes, such as fragrance mix, are useful to test larger numbers of allergens on the back; however, false positive reactions can occur with these mixes. The individual allergens in the mix, e.g. eight fragrance ingredients in fragrance mix, can then be tested separately to establish which exact allergens need to be avoided. If this further testing is negative this suggests a false positive reaction has occurred to the mix. Investigators should be aware of possible side effects with patch testing (Box 6.6).

Box 6.5: Allergen series available

- Bakery series
- Cosmetic series
- Epoxy series
- Fragrance series
- Hairdressing series
- Isocyanate series
- Leg ulcer series
- Methacrylate series (adhesives, dental and other)
- Methacrylate series (printing)
- Photographic chemicals series
- Plant series
- Rubber additives series
- Shoe series
- Textile colours and finish

Box 6.6: Side effects of patch testing

- Multiple severe reactions: 'angry back'
- Flare of existing dermatitis
- Pigment change
- Blistering/necrosis/scar
- Active sensitization

Treatment and patient education

Treatment of ACD consists of three steps:

1. Identify the relevant allergen.
2. Treat the current problem with topical or systemic treatment.
3. Educate the patient to avoid contact with these allergens.

Once relevant allergens are identified the patient should be given written information on all these chemicals. Complicating the information is the fact that many chemicals have numerous synonyms and can cross-react with other chemicals. The information sheets are available from books or commercially. Most departments have specific ones they use, and the British Contact Dermatitis Society has produced comprehensive up-to-date medical and patient information sheets for its standard series allergens. Information sheets are also available online from the British Association of Dermatologists at www.bad.org.uk.

OCCUPATIONAL CONTACT DERMATITIS

Occupational contact dermatitis can be caused by either an irritant (e.g. direct contact with caustic agents) or allergic contact (rubber glove allergy).

Irritant contact dermatitis (ICD) can be divided into several types.

Figure 6.4
(a) Positive patch test reactions shown on back. (b) 3+ (bullous) reaction to 4-phenylenediamine base (PPD).

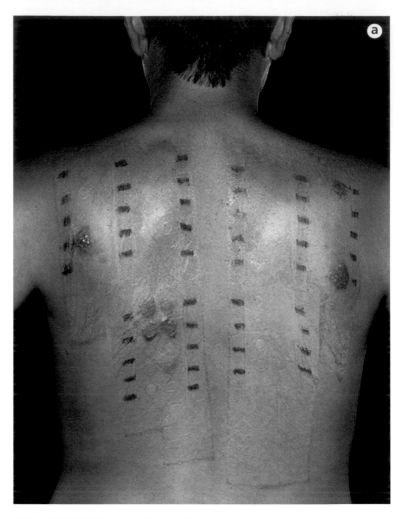

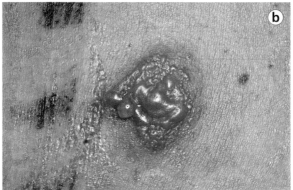

Acute ICD results from a single contact with a strong chemical substance causing an acute strong reaction similar to a burn.

Acute delayed ICD shows a delayed reaction with the irritant contact dermatitis developing 8–24 hours after the initial contact, for example dithranol reactions.

Irritant reaction ICD is a subclinical dermatitis common in hairdressers and metal workers, with a clinical picture of dermatitis starting under the rings and usually spreading over the dorsum of the hands.

Cumulative ICD is a result of repeated exposure to irritants such as soaps, shampoos, detergents and mild acids and alkalis. This can result in erythema, dryness and cracking and irritant hand dermatitis.

Pustular and acneiform ICD can follow exposure to oils, greases and tars. Atopics and previous acne sufferers are most prone.

The diagnosis of irritant contact dermatitis is usually made by exclusion of allergic contact dermatitis. The commonest manifestation of ICD is hand dermatitis which is discussed in detail later in this chapter.

Allergic contact dermatitis occurs much less frequently than ICD, but is of great importance as it can frequently force a worker to change jobs, as protective measures often fail to work. ACD must be differentiated from atopic dermatitis, psoriasis, pustular eruptions, herpes simplex and zoster infections, fungal infections and irritant contact dermatitis. Patch testing must be thorough as there may be unknown compounds and testing to the patients' own items is essential. Examples of allergens encountered in various occupations is shown below (Table 6.2).

Key points for patch tests

- Take a good contact and occupational history including hobbies.
- Decide on appropriate patch tests.
- Patch test to specific own items if allergy is suspected.
- Leave patches on back for 2 days.
- Final reading done at 4 days.
- Note any positive reactions and distinguish from irritant reactions.
- Give the patient the relevant information.

EXPERT WITNESSES AND MEDICOLEGAL REPORTS

Training in writing a few medicolegal reports is an essential requirement in the dermatology curriculum. In reality, this may be difficult for specialist registrars to achieve during their training period and usually involves shadowing a consultant who is involved with a current medicolegal report. This section will describe briefly the main points required to deal with the process of writing such a document (Box 6.7).

There are a number of courses available now providing training in report writing and how to be a medical expert witness in court. The expert witness (EW) must state their qualifications (e.g. degrees, courses, training, lecturing, publications) and their experience including time

Table 6.2: Examples of allergens encountered in various occupations

Occupations	Allergens
Agriculture workers	Rubber, oats, barley, animal feed, veterinary medications, cement, plants, pesticides, wood preservatives
Bakers and confectioners	Flavours and spices, orange, lemon, essential oils, dyes, ammonium persulphate and benzoyl peroxide
Bartenders	Orange, lemon, lime, flavours
Butchers	Nickel, sawdust
Cleaners	Rubber gloves
Construction workers	Chromates, cobalt, rubber and leather gloves, resins, woods
Cooks and caterers	Foods, onions, garlic, spices, flavours, rubber gloves, sodium metabisulphite, lauryl and octyl gallate, formaldehyde
Dentists and dental technicians	Local anesthetics, mercury, methacrylates, eugenol, disinfectants, rubber
Electricians	Fluxes, resins, rubber
Electroplaters	Nickel, chromium, cobalt
Embalmers	Formaldehyde
Florists and gardeners	Plants, pesticides, rubber gloves
Foundry workers	Phenol- and urea-formaldehyde resins, colophony
Hairdressers	Dyes, persulphates, nickel, perfumes, rubber gloves, formaldehyde
Homemakers	Rubber gloves, foods, spices, flavours, nickel, chromates, polishes
Jewellers	Epoxy resin, metals, soldering fluxes
Mechanics	Rubber gloves, chromates, epoxy resin, antifreeze
Medical personnel	Rubber gloves, anaesthetics, antibiotics, antiseptics, phenothiazines, formaldehyde, glutaraldehyde, chloroxylenol, hand creams
Metal workers	Nickel, chromates, additives in some cutting oils
Office workers	Rubber, nickel, glue
Painters	Turpentine, cobalt, chromates, polyester resins, formaldehyde, epoxy resin, adhesives, paints
Photography industry workers	Rubber gloves, colour developers, para-aminophenol, hydroquinone, formaldehyde, sodium metabisulphite, chromates
Plastic workers	Hardeners, phenolic resins, polyurethanes, acrylics, plasticizers
Printers	Nickel, chromates, cobalt, colophony, formaldehyde, turpentine
Rubber workers	Rubber chemicals, dyes, colophony
Shoemakers	Glues, leather, rubber, turpentine
Tannery workers	Chromates, formaldehyde, tanning agents, fungicides, dyes
Textile workers	Formaldehyde resins, dyes, chromates, nickel

Box 6.7: Medicolegal report contents

Introduction

- Specialist details
- Summary of case
- Summary of conclusions

The issues

Investigation of facts: history and examination

Opinion

Prognosis

Statement of compliance

Statement of fact

Appendices

- Documents examined (copies of important ones)
- Published references
- Photographs
- Glossary of technical/medical terms

spent in the area of expertise and their job appointments. The EW is an independent advisor and must understand their duty to the court and comply with that duty at all times. The EW aims to provide an opinion on facts in the field of expertise outside common knowledge.

The terms and conditions of engagement is the legal position between solicitors, expert witnesses and their clients. The solicitor usually engages the EW wherein they provide advice, report writing and court appearances if necessary. The solicitor is liable for the EW fees even if the client does not pay the solicitor and a prior letter of engagement is essential from the EW to the solicitor. Estimates of costs can be helpful for the solicitor and can be stated in this letter. If any tests are required, details of the person to perform these and the costs should be sent. Accurate records of time spent on the case need to be documented for reading of hospital files and general practitioner notes, client interview, possible factory visits and any research involved.

The new Civil Procedure Rules, part 35, effective from April 1999 are important. This aims to limit the use of oral expert evidence. A single expert witness may be involved with the case and the court's permission is required to call an expert or use an expert's report in evidence. Hence, the report should be addressed to the court and not to the engaging party, e.g. solicitor. Do not comment on any negligence as this is for the court to decide.

The basic content of the medicolegal report should define the issue and establish the facts with a detailed history and examination as relevant to the case. A basic layout is shown in Box 6.7. The issues should be stated clearly and briefly and could include causation (i.e what, why, where, how and when), responsibility (liability) or amount (e.g how much, how long). For a case of hand dermatitis this could include the cause of the dermatitis, whether this is permanent, possible successful treatment and the potential cost and length of treatment including the prognosis.

The facts include what has been observed, stated and recorded in documents. The facts need to be 100% accurate and nothing should be made up or guessed. Medical history and examination can include present details of the client with dates of entries in notes and any comments made by medical practitioners including treatments. If any facts are recalled or from memory of the patient then this should be clearly stated. Details of past medical history relevant to the case is important and the diagnosis or proposed diagnosis needs to be stated. The effect of the condition on continuation of current employment or on finding alternative employment should be included. If any documents are reviewed such as Material Safety Data Sheets, any relevant details can be highlighted such as chemicals possibly causing allergy or irritation.

An opinion is then expressed (in the first person) on the basis of those facts which deal with the issues identified. The lawyers will expect the opinions to have reasons, i.e 'because of …'. A statement of prognosis can be made, e.g. for hand dermatitis. Finally, statements of compliance (e.g. I understand that my duty in preparing this report is to the court and I have complied with that duty) and truth (e.g. I believe that the facts I have stated in this report are true and the opinions I have expressed are correct) need to be made. Where there is a range of opinion on matters dealt with in the report, a summary of the range of opinion and the reasons for the EW's own opinion must be stated.

A summary of the conclusions reached is required in the document which needs to be signed and dated. Appendices can be included of copies of relevant documents, literature and references quoted, glossary of medical terms, and photographs. General style should be easy to read and understand with short sentences and paragraphs. Avoid terms such as 'never' and 'always'. The presentation should be of high standard printed on quality paper with clear headings and well margined, numbered pages and paragraphs. Overall, the whole document should be easy for all parties concerned including judges and lawyers!

HAND DERMATITIS

Hand dermatitis is usually a manifestation of both irritant and allergic contact dermatitis although it can be caused by a number of other dermatitic eruptions of the hand such as atopic hand dermatitis. A suggested management plan is shown in Figure 6.5.

Hand protection with gloves

An increased awareness of the risks of developing irritant and allergic contact dermatitis in the home and the workplace has led to an increased interest in both the usage of gloves and adverse events related to wearing these gloves.

Protective gloves are one of the key elements in the management of primary and secondary contact dermatitis. The materials used for the manufacture of protective gloves are natural rubber, synthetic rubber, textile fibres, leather and several polymeric materials. The protective effect of these different glove materials is dependent on both the thickness of the glove and composition of these materials.

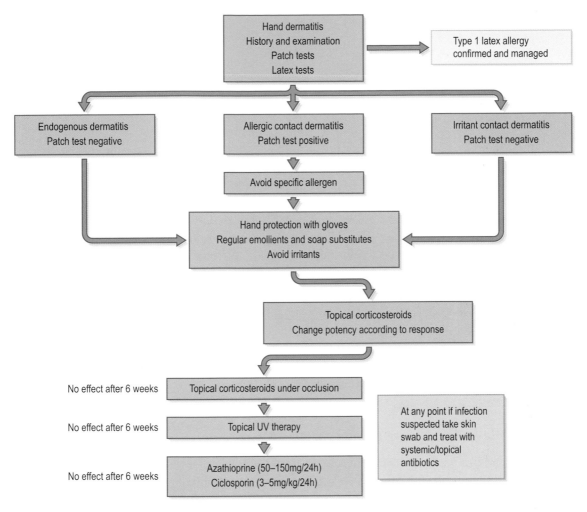

Figure 6.5
Management of hand dermatitis.

If the patient is to use gloves for domestic tasks such as washing dishes and clothes they should be asked to purchase plastic or PVC gloves rather than rubber since rubber can cause an allergic contact dermatitis. Indeed gloves are the commonest cause of rubber dermatitis; the allergen is usually a thiuram chemical added to natural rubber latex.

The patient should be informed that gloves should not be worn for more than 15–20 minutes at a time and that if water enters a glove it should be taken off immediately. The patient can help to minimize the effects of contaminants by turning the gloves inside out and rinsing them several times a week in hot running water before allowing them to dry completely.

The penetration (leakage) of chemicals refers to the flow through seams, pinholes and other imperfections. Gloves for industrial use are subject to tests to assess penetration and gloves for medical use are tested for leakage. However, when users take the gloves on and off during the course of a working day for changes in tasks, mealtimes etc., the chemicals covering the outside commonly contaminate the glove inner surface. This negates any benefits of glove usage and hastens the development of irritant or allergic contact dermatitis caused by the occlusive effect of the glove. The patient needs to be made aware of this problem and instructed that if the inside of the glove becomes contaminated with chemicals or soaps both gloves should be rinsed out immediately and left to dry inside out. The patient should be reminded that if the gloves develop a hole or tear they should be discarded immediately.

Cotton gloves can be used under plastic gloves to soak up sweat that would otherwise irritate the skin, although some authorities argue that this simply potentiates the occlusive effect of gloves on sweat. These cotton liners should only be worn a few times before they are washed. Cotton gloves can also be very useful for 'dry' household chores. The patient should be told to purchase several pairs of plastic and cotton gloves at a time for use in the kitchen, bathroom and at work. They should also be reminded to use heavy-duty fabric gloves when doing any gardening, 'do-it-yourself' and outdoor work and to wear gloves when outdoors in cold weather to prevent the hands drying, cracking and chapping.

The actual protection afforded by gloves depends also on manufacturing quality, glove thickness, concentration of contactant, the duration of contact and environmental temperature and humidity. It should also be remembered that the talcum powder (talc) used in many gloves is also a skin irritant. The potentially harmful effect of talc is even greater if latex gloves are 'powdered', as the talc absorbs latex enhancing the overall latex exposure and increasing the risk of allergy development.

Use of soap substitutes and moisturizers

'Normal' soap and water can be very irritating to the hands of a patient with dermatitis. Patients should be told that when washing their hands, either at work or at home, they should always use lukewarm (preferably running) water and a moisturizer as a soap substitute. They should be advised to dry the skin carefully with a clean towel and pay particular attention to the interdigital spaces where irritants can accumulate.

Moisturizers used as soap substitutes can either be a water-based paraffin containing cream such as Aqueous Cream BP or, for more heavy-duty uses, a paraffin-based Emulsifying Ointment. Conversely, and for ease of application and increased patient compliance, soap substitutes should be chosen so that they can also be used as moisturizers applied directly to the skin to form a protective layer.

Moisturizers are not only important in the treatment of established soap or detergent induced irritant contact dermatitis, but have also been shown to have a preventative role in the development of irritant dermatitis, both in experimental domestic situations and in real life work situations.

Ideally, the patient should be prescribed several large tubs of moisturizer/soap substitute, which can then be placed next to every sink both at home and at work. Smaller tubes to carry around in a bag or in the car should also be given. The patient can be instructed to use the soap substitute as a general moisturizer and be reminded that these products are safe to apply to all areas of the skin even in children. The patient should be instructed to apply them several times a day or whenever their skin feels dry or itchy.

Barrier creams are sometimes referred to as 'protective ointments' or 'invisible gloves'. They are designed to prevent or reduce the penetration and absorption of various hazardous materials into the skin and replace protective clothing in situations where personal protective equipment such as gloves, sleeves or faceguards cannot be safely or conveniently used.

While they are often used in the management of contact dermatitis, actual benefits have not been conclusively proven and indeed some authorities argue that they exacerbate rather then ameliorate the situation. They are therefore recommended only for use with low-grade irritants such as water, detergents and cutting oils.

Avoidance of irritants

Irritant contact dermatitis is the commonest cause of exogenous hand dermatitis. In a study of hand eczema in over 1900 patients in the Netherlands, half the cases were diagnosed as irritant contact dermatitis. Patients who are medical workers, caterers, cleaners and housekeepers are particularly at risk. Indeed anyone who in the course of their occupational or domestic tasks washes his or her hands frequently may develop hand dermatitis leading to the use in the past of such terms as 'housewife's eczema' or 'dishpan hands'.

Eliminating the cause (or more often causes) of irritant contact dermatitis is not easy. However, as endogenous factors such as constitutional hand dermatitis cannot be changed, it is clear that avoidance of irritants is of paramount importance.

The success of irritant avoidance depends greatly on the compliance of the patient. It is important to counsel the patient that systematic protection of the hands is important, and that avoidance of irritants plays a large part in this. It also has to be realistically assumed that for some patients it will be impossible to follow these instructions to the letter. For these patients, partial irritant avoidance is still better than none.

All patients should be given a hand care information sheet with key points (Box 6.8). The patient should be asked to read this carefully several times and to try to follow these guidelines as fastidiously as possible. The patient should be encouraged to use only the emollients and soap substitutes that have been prescribed, as over-the-counter products may contain many different irritants. In addition, direct contact with detergents and other cleansing agents must be avoided as these are strong irritants. The patient should measure

---

Box 6.8: Key points in hand care information sheet

- Protect your hands with gloves
- Use soap substitutes
- Avoid irritants
- Continue for at least 6 months

out washing powder and detergents carefully using only the amount recommended on the packaging and keep the outside of the packaging free of spillage to avoid direct contact with the detergents and cleansing agents. Skin cleansers used at work are also harsh on the hands and direct contact with these is best avoided altogether.

Soap and detergents may damage the skin by several mechanisms. Alkali-induced damage of the stratum corneum increases permeability of the horny layer, and removal of lipids and amino acids of the skin by soaps and detergents damages the water-holding capacity of the horny layer. In addition, certain components of soaps such as fatty acids may be directly irritant. For these reasons patients should be instructed to always use a soap substitute.

To avoid any prolonged contact with irritants, patients should also be instructed to use running water if possible when washing up and reminded that rings should not be worn at all during housework or other wet work even after their dermatitis has clinically disappeared and healed. Rings should be cleaned on the inside frequently with a brush then rinsed thoroughly and patients should not wash their hands with soap when wearing a ring. The use of washing machines and dishwashers is the ideal way to protect hands from irritants.

The patient should be provided with a list of irritants that need to be avoided in the domestic situation. This is important not only for those who perform traditional household tasks but also in more heavy-duty domestic chores such as car washing, painting and decorating. A list of potential irritants is given in Box 6.9.

It is important for the patient to be made familiar with these irritants and recognize where they are likely to come into contact with them, as this understanding will improve compliance. A full explanation by the physician is also more likely to improve compliance and therefore outcome.

Prognosis and ongoing management

It is good practice to give the patient realistic advice with respect to the prognosis of their hand dermatitis and the importance of continuing the above measures indefinitely. Many patients expect only to carry out these measures for the duration of the clinical disease and do not realize that their tendency to develop irritant hand dermatitis will be life-long especially if they have an atopic background.

It is important for the patient to consider any triggering events that may have been responsible for the initial appearance of an episode of hand dermatitis. Irritant dermatitis can appear for the first time after the birth of a child or when an elderly relative needing

Box 6.9: *Common skin irritants*

- Shampoos and conditioners
- Hair products such as hair lotions and hair dyes
- Polishes including metal, wax, shoe, floor, car, furniture and window polishes
- Solvents and stain-removers such as white spirit, petrol, trichloroethylene and turpentine
- Foods such as oranges, lemons, grapefruit, potatoes or tomatoes

care is taken in. Retirement with an increase in housework, maintenance or gardening duties can also precipitate hand dermatitis. The patient may associate these events with increased 'stress' and blame their skin condition on this.

The patient should be told that it will take some months for their skin to return to below the irritant threshold and for clinical dermatitis to disappear. We tell our patients that the skin will remain vulnerable for at least 6 months after the dermatitis appears to be completely healed so they have to continue to follow the above instructions. A minority of patients may continue to develop problems despite following this advice and will require more aggressive second line therapy as discussed later in this chapter. For those with an underlying atopic diathesis, especially those in occupations associated with a high risk of hand dermatitis such as nursing, we recommend that the hand care guidelines described above be followed indefinitely.

Treatment of hand dermatitis

Topical emollients and steroids are the mainstays in the treatment of hand dermatitis. A management algorithm is shown in Figure 6.5.

Emollients

Most hand dermatitis is characterized by dryness and scaling that will require regular re-application of moisturizers. The patient should be offered a selection of emollients with different characteristics. In general terms, the greasier the emollient the better its effect on dry skin, but the messier an emollient is, the less likely the patient is to apply it regularly. A useful compromise is to prescribe both a less greasy product such as Aqueous Cream BP for use in the morning and throughout the day and to prescribe an oilier emollient such as Emulsifying Ointment BP for use once the patient has finished the day's work. We offer our patients a number of different emollient samples to try out both in the clinic and at home in order to strike a balance between the emollient needs of the skin and what is acceptable to the individual patient, thus optimizing compliance.

Corticosteroids

Topical corticosteroids

Topical corticosteroids are often one of the key elements in treating patients with hand dermatitis. Issues to consider when assessing the patient include whether to treat with cream or ointment and what strength of topical steroid to use. Most corticosteroid creams are insufficiently lubricating but corticosteroid ointments, the clinicians' preferred option, may be unacceptably greasy to some patients and again a balance must be struck to increase compliance.

Different hand sites respond differently to the same strength of topical steroids. The choice of topical corticosteroid therapy depends on the location and severity of the dermatitis. Dermatitis of the back of the hands responds more readily than palmar dermatitis due to the differences in stratum corneum thickness. Frequent use of a potent topical steroid may

109

cause cutaneous atrophy. Whether topical steroids should be used once or more frequently every day, and whether short bursts of topical steroids are preferable to constant treatment, have not yet been directly addressed in studies of patients with hand dermatitis.

In a randomized, double blind, parallel group study to determine whether a 3-day burst of a potent corticosteroid is more effective than a mild preparation used for 7 days in children with mild or moderate atopic eczema, no differences were found between the two groups. Therefore a short burst of a potent topical corticosteroid is just as effective as prolonged use of a milder preparation for controlling mild or moderate atopic eczema in children.

In patients unresponsive to standard regimens, the effectiveness of topical therapy can be increased by occlusion. Plastic occlusion increases corticosteroid penetration approximately ten-fold. In hand dermatitis occlusion can lead to rapid healing of fissures and dramatically improves psoriasiform and atopic hand dermatitis. Unfortunately it also increases the risk of unwanted side effects such as skin atrophy especially if combined with super potent steroids. Occlusion of the hands is best accomplished by wearing thin plastic (not rubber) gloves overnight. This technique is initially uncomfortable to the patient, but is very beneficial after a few days. In patients with low grade but very dry hand dermatitis emollients alone can be used under occlusion to improve their efficacy.

Systemic corticosteroids

In acute, severe, blistering hand dermatitis, a brief course of systemic corticosteroids often has a dramatic effect. The aim is to improve the dermatitis sufficiently for topical treatment to be effective. One recommended regimen is to use a 10 day tapering course of prednisolone, starting at 40 mg and reducing by 5 mg each day. Topical corticosteroids should be added as soon as the blistering and oedema starts to decrease.

Topical and systemic antibiotics

Hand dermatitis can become secondarily infected and require recurrent courses of oral antibiotics. Some clinicians prefer a systemic antibiotic and a topical corticosteroid although there is some evidence for the efficacy of topical antibiotic and corticosteroid combination treatment in atopic and contact dermatitis.

Topical antiseptic soaks such as potassium permanganate are useful in acutely inflamed or infected hand dermatitis where they help to combat infection and in acute blistering hand dermatitis where they help to dry up the hands. Important practical issues include taking skin swabs for culture and sensitivity to determine appropriate antibiotic therapy.

Photochemotherapy

Psoralen ultraviolet A (PUVA) treatment is a useful option for unresponsive hand dermatitis, where psoralen is taken either orally or the hands are soaked in psoralen solution prior to the UVA treatment. In a left-right comparison of ultraviolet B (UVB) phototherapy and topical photochemotherapy (PUVA) in bilateral chronic hand dermatitis for 6 weeks, no significant differences in improvement were demonstrated between the modalities, but side effects occurred more often on the PUVA-treated side. This treatment modality is discussed in more detail in Chapter 10.

Systemic immunosuppressants

Ciclosporin has been shown to be effective in the management of hand dermatitis. In a comparison study in the treatment of severe chronic hand dermatitis, ciclosporin at 3 mg/kg/day was as effective as topical betamethasone-17, 21-dipropionate. Low-dose ciclosporin is a useful additional treatment for the short-term treatment of severe chronic hand dermatitis in patients unresponsive to conventional therapy but is contraindicated in patients with hypertension or renal disease and requires regular, careful monitoring of blood electrolytes and blood pressure.

Azathioprine can be used to establish control of atopic dermatitis although no controlled studies have been performed in hand dermatitis and it can take more than 4 weeks to be effective. In a double blind, randomized, placebo-controlled, crossover trial of azathioprine in adult patients with severe atopic dermatitis, there was significant improvement in the active treatment group compared to placebo. This improvement must be balanced against the drug's hepatotoxicity, potential for bone marrow suppression and gastrointestinal side effects, and therapy requires regular monitoring of the full blood count and liver enzymes.

Topical immunosuppressives

Tacrolimus ointment has been shown to have some beneficial effect in long-standing cases of chronic dyshidrotic palmar eczema, and further emerging topical immunosuppressive drugs may prove to be very helpful in the future management of hand dermatitis.

Further reading

Bourke J, Coulson I, English J. Guidelines for care of contact dermatitis. Br J Dermatol 2001; 145:877–885.

Britton JER, Wilkinson SM, English JSC, et al. The British Standard Series of contact dermatitis allergens: validation in clinical practice and value for clinical governance. Br J Dermatol 2003; 148:259–264.

Chowdhury MMU, Maibach HI. Occupational skin disorders. In: LaDou J, ed. Current occupational and environmental medicine. 3rd edn. New York: Lange; 2003:287–306.

Chowdhury MMU, Statham BN, Sansom JE, et al. Patch testing for corticosteroid allergy with low and high concentrations of tixocortol pivalate and budesonide. Contact Dermatitis 2002; 46:311–312.

Chowdhury MMU, Statham BN. Natural rubber latex allergy in a Welsh healthcare population. Br J Dermatol 2003; 148:737–740.

Johnston GA, Nicolaou N, Chowdhury MMU. Management of hand dermatitis. In: Chowdhury MMU, Maibach HI, eds. Latex intolerance: basic science, epidemiology and clinical management. Boca Raton, FL: CRC Press; 2005:151–164.

Katugampola RP, Statham BN, English JSC, et al. A multicentre review of footwear allergens tested in the United Kingdom. Contact Dermatitis 2005; 53:133–135.

Katugampola RP, Statham BN, English JSC, et al. A multicentre review of hairdressing allergens tested in the United Kingdom. Contact Dermatitis 2005; 53:130–132.

Lewis VJ, Statham BN, Chowdhury MMU. Allergic contact dermatitis in 191 consecutively patch-tested children. Contact Dermatitis 2004; 51:155–156.

Zhai H, Chowdhury MMU, Maibach HI. Barrier creams/moisturizers. In: Chowdhury MMU, Maibach HI, eds. Latex intolerance: basic science, epidemiology and clinical management. Boca Raton, FL: CRC Press; 2005:165–176.

Introductory textbooks

Lachapelle J-M, Maibach HI, eds. Patch testing and prick testing: a practical guide. Berlin: Springer; 2003.

Wahlberg JE, Elsner P, Kanerva L, Maibach HI, eds. Management of positive patch test reactions. Berlin: Springer; 2003.

Reference textbooks

Kanerva L, Elsner P, Wahlberg JE, Maibach HI, eds. Handbook of occupational dermatology. Berlin: Springer; 2000.

Rietschel RL, Fowler JF, eds. Fisher's contact dermatitis. Philadelphia: Lippincott Williams & Wilkins; 2001.

Rycroft RJG, Menne T, Frosch PJ, Lepoittevin J-P, eds. Textbook of contact dermatitis. Berlin: Springer; 2001.

Useful websites

http://orgs.dermis.net/content/ (European Contact Dermatitis Societies)

www.bcds.org.uk (British Contact Dermatitis Society)

www.blackwellpublishing.com (Contact Dermatitis and other journals)

www.chemotechnique.se (Chemotechnique allergens)

www.contactderm.org (American Contact Dermatitis Society)

www.hermal.de (Trolab allergens)

www.occmed.oxfordjournals.org (Occupational Medicine journal)

Systemic therapy

7

Richard E. A. Williams

INTRODUCTION

The development of effective systemic therapies has enhanced the dermatologist's ability to help patients with severe and disabling dermatoses. While the benefits to patients can be great, systemic agents demand complex prescribing skills and careful monitoring. This chapter endeavours to explore some of these themes but does not attempt to be comprehensive. It concentrates on drugs used frequently in dermatology and on those in which careful monitoring is necessary. Particularly with new or unfamiliar drugs, the prescriber is directed to standard references such as the British National Formulary, Martindale:The Complete Drug Reference and Comprehensive Dermatologic Drug Therapy. An important recent addition is the British National Formulary for Children. New editions of these publications are produced regularly and some on-line versions can be accessed via the NHS net. Guidelines produced by learned bodies and each drug's summary of product characteristics (available on-line in the electronic medicine compendium) are also valuable, up-to-date sources of information. Discussions with one's peers and other healthcare professionals such as pharmacists are always helpful.

GENERAL CONSIDERATIONS

Prescribing systemic therapy

Prescribing is a complicated process. The approach is centred on the individual patient but can be conveniently broken down into patient factors, prescriber factors, the dermatological condition to be treated, the proposed drug to be prescribed and external factors (Box 7.1). Careful consideration of each of these is required on every occasion and the end result should be considered a contract of care between the patient and physician.

While prescribing is based on evidence, every time a patient takes a drug it is in effect a clinical experiment with only a partially predictable outcome. Systemic therapy can sometimes be life saving. In dermatology however, the majority of patients, whilst suffering significant impairment of quality of life, will not be generally unwell. In this group of

---

Box 7.1: *Examples of factors to consider when prescribing systemic therapy*

Patient

- Patient preferences
- Age, sex
- Social circumstances including employment
- Co-morbidity and past medical history
- Medication history

Prescriber factors

- Knowledge
- Experience
- Previous critical incidents
- Prescribing bias

Dermatological condition

- Severity
- Treatment guidelines
- Expected response to proposed treatment

Proposed systemic therapy

- Efficacy
- Route of administration
- Dose and formulation
- Pharmacogenetics
- Toxicity
- Cost
- Licence status

External factors

- Clinical governance (e.g. NICE, guidelines, protocols, licensing authorities)
- Financial

---

patients it is therefore particularly important to consider benefit:risk ratios. Remember Hippocrates' bidding to 'First, do no harm'.

Increasingly, the direct doctor–patient prescribing environment is being influenced by external factors. These include clinical governance issues and financial constraints. Prescribers need to be aware of both local and national policies and frameworks (e.g. National Institute for Clinical Excellence (NICE) guidelines, formularies and local Drugs and Therapeutics committees).

Patient information leaflets

Information leaflets serve many useful purposes. They facilitate informed consent by explaining what may be expected from the treatment and by documenting potential adverse reactions. They should also provide outline schedules for monitoring so that the patient can be encouraged to take some ongoing responsibility. Patient information leaflets are readily available from bodies such as the British Association of Dermatologists.

Guidelines and protocols

Aide memoirs such as guidelines and protocols contribute to comprehensive assessments, high quality of care, audit and nurse-led monitoring. A treatment initiation sheet including tick boxes with regards to indications, contraindications and monitoring can be particularly helpful. Deviation from guidelines and protocols may be appropriate in the individual patient but the prescriber should always be prepared to justify such action.

Drug monitoring

Both the initial and continuing prescribers bear the responsibility to ensure that appropriate monitoring is undertaken. This may occur either entirely in secondary care, completely in primary care or increasingly through the concept of shared care. In shared care, monitoring is usually protocol driven with the option of patient held records to facilitate information exchange between patient, general practitioner, consultant and specialist nurse. As part of the process of monitoring, attention should be paid not only to absolute values of measured parameters but also to trends within reference ranges.

Combination therapy

There may be a variety of reasons for prescribing drugs in combination. One may simply be trying to produce cumulative benefit. Alternatively, by using lower doses of one or both drugs one can attempt to achieve the desired therapeutic effect but with lower toxicity. It is generally wise to start off with one drug and to add a second initially at a low dose and increase slowly with careful monitoring. Specific drug interactions are well documented in the British National Formulary.

Unlicensed drugs and 'off label' prescribing of licensed drugs

Doctors are free to prescribe both unlicensed drugs and also licensed drugs outside of their product licence (so called 'off label'). This is a frequent scenario in dermatology. Prescribers must be aware that in these situations their personal responsibility is increased. In the event of an adverse reaction they should be in a position to demonstrate that they have acted with reasonable care and skill. The patient should be told of the unlicensed status of the prescription and best practice would be to make a written note of the discussion to document informed consent. Consultants should be prepared to be supportive and provide information if requests are made to general practitioners to prescribe in an unlicensed situation. For a more detailed discussion of this subject the reader is directed to Drugs and Therapeutics Bulletin 1992; 30(25):97–99.

Prescribing for children

Children are not simply small adults. Drugs may be handled differently, particularly in the neonate. Doses are calculated on body weight or body surface area. The new British National Formulary for Children is an invaluable source of information.

INDIVIDUAL DRUGS

Guidelines on the use of individual drugs are produced by societies such as the British Association of Dermatologists, Royal College of Physicians and the American Academy of Dermatology. These are valuable contemporary sources of information. Recommendations for doses, monitoring, etc. often vary between authorities. Any regimens suggested in this chapter should be verified against other publications and tailored to each individual patient. Only certain aspects of each drug will be discussed and the reader is again directed to larger reference works for further details.

Systemic steroids

The introduction of systemic corticosteroids was a major advance in dermatology. Whilst new agents continue to be developed, corticosteroids remain an indispensable tool in dermatological practice. The most frequently used systemic corticosteroid is oral prednisolone. Others include hydrocortisone, methylprednisolone and dexamethasone.

Mechanisms of action

Corticosteroids act on intracellular glucocorticoid receptors to produce a myriad of actions. The end results are anti-inflammatory, antiproliferative, immunosuppressive and the production of vasoconstriction. Each of the different corticosteroids has a glucocorticoid component and most, except dexamethasone, mineralocorticoid activity as well (Table 7.1).

Formulations, doses and duration

Systemic steroids may be given orally, intravenously and rarely, intramuscularly.

Oral route

While prednisolone has a plasma half-life of up to 4 hours, it is biologically active for 24 to 36 hours. The drug is therefore usually given as a once daily dose first thing in the morning. This is to minimize the suppressive effect of the exogenous corticosteroid on the pituitary adrenal axis. Doses vary greatly between diseases and patients. Starting doses rarely exceed 1 mg/kg/day but are more typically 0.5 mg/kg/day. Duration and reduction in dose also vary widely, although tapering is usually needed to avoid disease flares. The general principle is to use the least dose necessary to suppress the disease and to use it for the minimum period of time. When disease activity has been controlled, alternate day treatment is an option in

Table 7.1: Comparison of corticosteroids	
	Equivalent anti-inflammatory dose
Prednisolone	5 mg
Hydrocortisone	20 mg
Methylprednisolone	4 mg
Dexamethasone	0.75 mg

an attempt to reduce adrenal suppression. The switch from once daily treatment should be done gradually however to minimize the chances of a flare of the disease.

Dexamethasone has insignificant mineralocorticoid activity. It can therefore be a useful option where high doses of prednisolone are required but fluid retention would be problematic. It is long acting (plasma half life 2 to 5 hours, biological half-life 36 to 54 hours).

Intravenous route

Hydrocortisone, which is short acting (plasma half-life 1 to 2 hours, biological half-life up to 12 hours), is useful intravenously for emergencies such as anaphylaxis and where there is short term inability to take oral medication, e.g. perioperatively.

Methylprednisolone is given by intravenous infusion at a dose of 500 mg to 1 gm daily for 5 days ('pulsed therapy') in an attempt to produce faster onset of therapeutic effect, usually in patients with severe or refractory disease. It carries with it an increased risk from sudden death (presumed to be cardiac), electrolyte shift, thromboembolic disease and psychosis.

Intramuscular route

Regular intramuscular injections are painful and mostly unnecessary. A depot preparation of methylprednisolone 40–120 mg may be useful intramuscularly when concordance with oral therapy is a problem. The main disadvantage is that because of the depot nature of the preparation the drug cannot be withdrawn quickly if adverse effects occur.

Monitoring and side effects

Systemic steroids have a wide spectrum of adverse effects (Figure 7.1). Those requiring ongoing monitoring include hyperglycaemia, hypertension, weight gain, and in children, growth retardation.

The risk of gastrointestinal bleeding with systemic steroids is greatest when co-prescribed with non-steroidal anti-inflammatory drugs (NSAIDs) including aspirin. In these circumstances, prophylaxis with proton pump inhibitors such as omeprazole should be considered, especially in the elderly. There is no advantage in using 'enteric coated' preparations as the effect of prednisolone on the gastrointestinal tract is mediated systemically rather than locally.

The elderly are also particularly susceptible to corticosteroid induced osteoporosis. Current recommendations from the Royal College of Physicians of London are that all patients over the age of 65 years expected to receive steroids for longer than 6 weeks should receive prophylaxis usually in the form of bisphosphonates started early in the course. Younger patients are usually managed on the basis of serial bone densitometry estimations but the limited availability of this investigation can cause practical difficulties.

Interactions

Corticosteroids antagonize the therapeutic effect of a number of drugs including hypotensives, hypoglycaemics and diuretics. Their use also increases the risk of gastrointestinal haemorrhage when given with NSAIDs. Anticoagulants may be either potentiated or inhibited although high doses of corticosteroids usually enhance the anticoagulant effect. The haematological toxicity of methotrexate is increased by

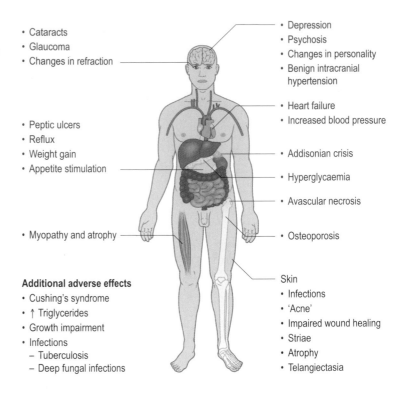

Figure 7.1
The side effects of corticosteroids extend to every body system.

- Cataracts
- Glaucoma
- Changes in refraction

- Depression
- Psychosis
- Changes in personality
- Benign intracranial hypertension

- Heart failure
- Increased blood pressure

- Peptic ulcers
- Reflux
- Weight gain
- Appetite stimulation

- Addisonian crisis
- Hyperglycaemia
- Avascular necrosis

- Myopathy and atrophy

- Osteoporosis

Skin
- Infections
- 'Acne'
- Impaired wound healing
- Striae
- Atrophy
- Telangiectasia

Additional adverse effects
- Cushing's syndrome
- ↑ Triglycerides
- Growth impairment
- Infections
  – Tuberculosis
  – Deep fungal infections

corticosteroids. High doses of corticosteroids reduce the immune response to vaccines and therefore live vaccines should be avoided.

Discontinuation of systemic corticosteroid therapy

Courses of corticosteroids of longer than 3 weeks may produce pituitary–adrenal suppression. Withdrawal from treatment should therefore usually be gradual, particularly after reaching the physiological level of 7.5 mg once daily of prednisolone.

Methotrexate

The main indication for methotrexate is in the management of pustular, erythrodermic or resistant chronic plaque psoriasis. It can also be effective in a proportion of patients with a large range of inflammatory dermatoses including sarcoidosis and lupus erythematosus.

Mechanisms of action

The long held view was that methotrexate exerted its therapeutic effect by inhibiting dihydrofolate reductase, thereby suppressing epidermal proliferation. Evidence now points more towards an immunological mode of action via an effect on lymphocytes.

Formulations, doses and duration

Most patients are maintained on oral methotrexate at a dose of between 5 mg and 25 mg once weekly. Intravenous, intramuscular and subcutaneous routes are also possible but are rarely necessary in dermatological practice. Initiation of treatment requires special care and most practitioners would use an initial test dose of 2.5 mg or 5 mg to assess potential idiosyncratic sensitivity. This is particularly important in the elderly. After the test dose has been successfully given the alternatives are to gradually increase the dose on a weekly basis or to immediately prescribe what is felt to be likely to be the maintenance dose, e.g. 10 mg once weekly. In pustular and erythrodermic psoriasis one often sees a response within a few doses whilst chronic plaque psoriasis may improve only after 6–8 weeks. Once control of the disease has been achieved then a gradual reduction in dose is indicated although the clinical effect of dose alterations at intervals of less than a month is difficult to assess.

Monitoring and side effects

The major adverse effects of methotrexate are nausea, acute mucositis, marrow suppression, hepatotoxicity and rarely, pulmonary fibrosis.

Various techniques may help methotrexate induced nausea. Firstly, the once weekly dose can be split with each half being taken 12 hours apart. Secondly, the co-prescribing of folic acid 5 mg once daily may be helpful. Thirdly, ondansetron 8 mg 2 hours prior to the weekly methotrexate dose with further doses afterwards if necessary can be tried.

Mucosal ulceration is a sign of absolute or relative over-dosage. It may be accompanied by myelosuppression and even cutaneous necrosis. Rescue treatment with folinic acid is vital.

Much has been written and debated about the hepatotoxic effects of methotrexate. The effect is cumulative but no method of monitoring is completely satisfactory. Although there is no long term prospective comparative study, the potential for hepatotoxicity appears to be more of a problem in patients with psoriasis than those with rheumatoid arthritis for whom methotrexate is also a standard treatment. The gold standard of monitoring for hepatotoxicity is considered to be serial liver biopsy. This is important if there is any suggestion of pre-existing liver damage but many authorities argue that the morbidity and cost of regular liver biopsy is unnecessary. One cannot rely solely on liver function tests but regular assessment of procollagen 3 propeptide (PC3P) appears to be encouraging. Maintenance of low levels of PC3P provides some reassurance but the interpretation of elevated levels is difficult as they may be caused by a variety of inflammatory or fibrotic processes which are not specific to liver damage. High alcohol intake increases the chances of methotrexate toxicity.

Bone marrow suppression may be either acute or chronic. Its likelihood is increased by folate deficiency. Baseline estimation of full blood count and haematinic levels are essential and full blood count should be estimated weekly during the initiation phase of therapy but once stable doses are achieved this can be extended to every 2 to 3 months. It is important that trends in values as well as absolute levels are monitored to detect the earliest signs of potential toxicity.

Pulmonary fibrosis may rarely occur during methotrexate treatment. A baseline chest X-ray may be useful to compare any potential future change.

Methotrexate is excreted by the kidneys. If renal function becomes impaired, previous therapeutic doses may become toxic. Regular long term monitoring of renal function is therefore indicated.

Interactions

Aspirin, non-steroidal anti-inflammatory drugs, ciclosporin and probenecid increase methotrexate levels by decreasing renal clearance. Sulphonamides, trimethoprim and phenytoin increase methotrexate's anti-folate activity.

Contraceptive precautions

Women of child bearing age should take adequate contraceptive measures whilst taking methotrexate and for at least one menstrual cycle after treatment cessation. Methotrexate is also excreted in the breast milk and is therefore a contraindication to breastfeeding. General advice to men is that they should have ceased methotrexate for 3 months before fathering children.

Pharmaceutical considerations

Correct prescribing is vital in methotrexate management as deaths have occurred when simple errors have been made. Methotrexate is supplied in both 10 mg and 2.5 mg tablets. To avoid confusion and to allow for fine dose adjustment only prescribe 2.5 mg tablets. If folic acid is co-prescribed it is vital that the patient realizes that the physical appearance of the two tablets is very similar (Figure 7.2) as confusion could be catastrophic. The National Patient Safety Agency of the UK National Health Service has introduced a mandatory scheme of patient information leaflets and monitoring booklets (www.npsa.nhs.uk).

Ciclosporin

The introduction of ciclosporin into dermatological use added a valuable and, in particular, fast acting drug to the management of psoriasis, atopic dermatitis and a vast array of other inflammatory dermatoses such as pyoderma gangrenosum and chronic idiopathic urticaria. Its use requires careful monitoring.

Mechanisms of action

Ciclosporin acts mainly on helper T cells with particular inhibitory effects on the production of IL-2.

Figure 7.2
Folic acid and methotrexate tablets are easily confused, particularly by anybody with failing sight.

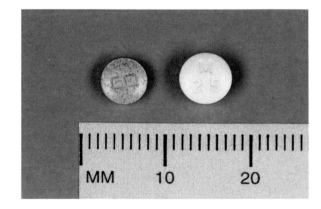

Formulations, doses and duration

Ciclosporin is usually administered orally on a twice daily basis. An intravenous preparation is also available. Different brands of oral ciclosporin preparations have markedly different bioavailabilities and therefore in the United Kingdom prescribing should be by brand name rather than generic.

The initial dose is usually between 3 mg and 5 mg/kg/day with subsequent tapering according to the clinical response. Treatment is best given in short intermittent courses of no more than 3 months at any time to avoid renal toxicity. Practically, this can often be difficult to implement as patients often achieve such a good response that they are loathe to stop treatment!

Monitoring and side effects

The main side effects of ciclosporin are nephrotoxicity and hypertension. At the initiation of treatment, at least two estimations of serum creatinine should be obtained and the average calculated. In patients with significant co-morbidities, such as cardiac failure, estimation of the glomerular filtration rate is advisable. The aim of monitoring thereafter is to contain any rise in serum creatinine to less than 130% of the patient's own average baseline creatinine. Initially, monitoring is required every 2 weeks but the time interval can be lengthened later on in any course. Likewise, at least two estimates of blood pressure should be obtained before treating and dose adjustment or concomitant antihypertensive treatment should be instigated if levels rise to the hypertensive range. Nifedipine should be avoided as an anti-hypertensive drug as in combination with ciclosporin it can cause very troublesome gum hypertrophy. Estimation of ciclosporin levels are not required when doses less than 5 mg/kg/day are prescribed as the necessary dose of ciclosporin can be judged by the clinical response and any potential nephrotoxicity or hypertensive tendency by direct measurement of these parameters. Other troublesome side effects, particularly early on in treatment, include nausea, peripheral dysaesthesia and hypertrichosis. It is also recommended to measure liver function tests, full blood count, serum lipids and serum urate during the initiation phase of ciclosporin therapy.

Interactions

A large number of interactions with ciclosporin are documented in the British National Formulary. Notable ones are the macrolide antibiotics, which increase plasma concentration of ciclosporin, non-steroidal anti-inflammatory drugs which can increase the nephrotoxicity, rifampicin which decreases the plasma concentration and finally grapefruit juice which increases the ciclosporin concentration in the plasma.

Hydroxycarbamide (hydroxyurea)

Hydroxycarbamide is a useful alternative therapy in psoriasis where it can be effective in up to 40% of patients. It can be used in situations where both methotrexate and ciclosporin are contraindicated.

Mechanism of action

Hydroxycarbamide inhibits ribonucleatide reductase preventing DNA synthesis and repair. This produces immunosuppression and radiation sensitization.

Formulations, doses and duration

Hydroxycarbamide is only available as an oral treatment. It is administered in doses starting at 500 mg once daily with potential increases to 1 gram and 1.5 grams daily. As long as careful monitoring is in place, there is no specific upper limit of duration of treatment. The drug may take a number of weeks to be effective in psoriasis.

Monitoring and side effects

The major adverse effect of hydroxycarbamide is marrow suppression. Full blood count needs to be monitored weekly during the initial 1 to 2 months of treatment with a decrease in the frequency of monitoring once the dose is stable. Dose reassessment should be triggered not only by values of haemoglobin, white cells and platelets below the reference range but also by downward trends within the reference range.

Recently, a dermatomyositis-like reaction has been described with hydroxycarbamide and it may also be responsible for seemingly intractable ulceration of the leg.

Azathioprine

Azathioprine is an anti-proliferative immunosuppressant. It can be used alone but is most often prescribed in combination with prednisolone.

Mechanism of action

Azathioprine is converted in vivo to 6-mercaptopurine which inhibits purine synthesis and acts as an immunosuppressant. Further metabolites may also be involved in the overall effect of azathioprine.

Formulations, doses and duration

Azathioprine is usually prescribed orally. Doses range between 1 mg and 3 mg/kg/day but typically are between 2 mg and 2.5 mg/kg/day. A very irritant alkaline intravenous preparation is available for emergency use but should be used only if the oral route is not possible. It is now recommended that before commencing azathioprine therapy the patient's thiopurine methyltransferase (TPMT) should be estimated. This enzyme is involved in the metabolism of azathioprine. Patients with low levels (less than 6 nmol/gHb/hr) should not receive azathioprine. Patients with so called 'carrier' levels of this enzyme (between 6 and 34 nmol/gHb/hr) should only receive azathioprine in reduced doses and with careful monitoring. The onset of action of azathioprine is between 6 and 12 weeks with the duration of treatment dependent upon the clinical situation. The haematological effect of azathioprine remains for about 1 month after stopping the drug whilst its immunological effect lasts for considerably longer, perhaps up to 2 to 3 months.

Monitoring and side effects

The major toxicities of azathioprine are myelosuppression and an allergic hepatitis. Full blood count and liver function tests should be tested at baseline and weekly for the first 4 weeks of treatment. The frequency of estimation can then be extended as indicated.

Azathioprine toxicity can occur unexpectedly and after seemingly prolonged periods of stability. In patients on azathioprine for many years following transplantation there is an increased risk of lymphoproliferative malignancy and squamous cell carcinomas of the skin.

Mycophenolate mofetil

Another drug inherited from renal transplant work, mycophenolate mofetil, is increasingly being used in auto-immune bullous disorders, psoriasis and atopic dermatitis. It is also useful as a steroid sparing agent.

Mechanism and action

Mycophenolate mofetil acts by inhibiting purine synthesis. This inhibition is particularly noticeable in lymphocytes.

Formulations, doses and duration

The oral route is the preferred one with doses starting at 500 mg twice daily and being increased according to the clinical response to a maximum of 2 grams twice daily. The onset of action may be delayed for up to 2–3 months. Duration of treatment is very variable depending upon the clinical situation.

Monitoring and side effects

Potential bone marrow suppression should be monitored by baseline full blood count, weekly blood counts for the first 4 weeks, twice a month for 2 months and then every month in the first year. Gastrointestinal effects such as nausea and diarrhoea are dose dependent.

Interactions

The absorption of mycophenolate mofetil is reduced by concurrent treatment with antacids and cholestyramine. There is an increased risk of agranulocytosis when mycophenolate is co-prescribed with clozapine.

Retinoids

The systemic retinoids available in the United Kingdom are isotretinoin, acitretin and bexarotene. They all represent chemical variations of retinol. Acitretin is used mostly in the treatment of psoriasis and isotretinoin in acne. Bexarotene is a recently introduced drug which can be helpful in some patients with cutaneous T-cell lymphoma. All three retinoids are fiercely teratogenic and in the United Kingdom there are licence restrictions (see individual 'summary of product characteristics' for details). There are no restrictions on males taking isotretinoin or acitretin concerning the fathering of children.

Mechanism of action

Retinoids act via specific receptors to produce effects on differentiation, tumour growth and neutrophil migration. Isotretinoin produces a major shrinking of sebaceous glands and a decrease in sebum production.

Formulations, doses and duration

Systemic retinoids are only available orally.

Isotretinoin

Isotretinoin is used mostly in the treatment of severe acne or acne resistant to other treatments. While the initial dose may be 0.5 mg/kg/day, the most efficacious regimen is 1.0 mg/kg/day for 16 weeks. Care needs to be exercised early on in a course of isotretinoin treatment particularly if the acne is severe and inflamed or if there are large numbers of macro-comedones. In severe and inflamed acne, pre-treatment with the combination of systemic prednisolone (0.5 mg/kg/day) and erythromycin (500 mg bd) should be considered. Once the inflammation has subsided, isotretinoin can then be added, initially at a low dose, gradually building up to the desired level. The prednisolone and erythromycin are tapered down depending on the clinical response. Macro-comedones should be treated with light cautery prior to the onset of isotretinoin therapy.

It is usual for isotretinoin to be effective in acne. Two thirds of patients receiving a 16 week course of 1 mg/kg/day do not require any further treatment of their acne. In the other third, recurrence may occur any time necessitating a second course. Occasionally patients require multiple courses.

Acitretin

The main indication for acitretin is psoriasis. It can be particularly effective in the pustular and acral varieties and when combined with PUVA. It is also used in a wide variety of disorders of keratinization such as Darier's disease or the ichthyoses. Long-term or intermittent treatment is required. Acitretin may be used in some skin malignancies such as cutaneous T-cell lymphoma but it can be particularly useful in transplant patients with multiple keratoses and squamous cell carcinomas.

The initial dose is usually 25 mg to 35 mg/day which can be increased to a maximum of 75 mg/day if required. Duration of therapy is very much dependent on the response.

Bexarotene

Bexarotene is a useful second line drug for the treatment of cutaneous T-cell lymphoma. The usual dose is 300 mg/m^2 body surface area/day.

Contraceptive precautions, side effects and monitoring

Isotretinoin, acitretin and bexarotene are all teratogenic. Females should not be pregnant at the initiation of retinoid therapy and should not become pregnant whilst taking it or after its cessation for 1 month in the case of isotretinoin and 2 years in the case of acitretin. Elaborate pregnancy prevention programmes have recently been developed in Europe for isotretinoin and all prescribers should be fully conversant with the information produced by the individual manufacturers of isotretinoin.

Nearly all patients taking retinoids develop mucocutaneous side effects. Cheilitis and dryness of the nasal vestibule are almost universal. These can be ameliorated with the use of emollients and topical steroids. Liver function tests should be monitored and fasting lipids measured at baseline and after about a month as very high serum triglycerides have been reported which could predispose the patient to acute pancreatitis.

When long-term acitretin is used, serum triglycerides should be monitored every 4–6 months. There is also a risk of diffuse idiopathic skeletal hypertrophy (DISH): monitoring regimens for this have not been standardized but it seems appropriate to X-ray the lumbar spine/sacroiliac joints once every 2–3 years.

A number of other side effects have been reported with the retinoids and special mention should be made of the possibility of mood changes and depression with isotretinoin. There are convincing anecdotal reports including suicides but population studies have failed to confirm overall increased risk. Nevertheless, all patients should be informed of the possible risk and the warning adequately documented.

Bexarotene is an emerging drug which can produce severe problems with hypothyroidism and hyperlipidaemia. Prescribers are referred to the 'summary of product characteristics' for details of the close monitoring that is required.

Interactions

Retinoids should not be prescribed with vitamin A supplements as this would lead to an increased risk of toxicity. There is an increased risk of benign intracranial hypertension when retinoids are prescribed with tetracyclines. Acitretin increases the concentration of methotrexate and concomitant use should generally be avoided because of an increased risk of hepatotoxicity.

Dapsone

The licensed indications for dapsone in the United Kingdom include treatment of leprosy and dermatitis herpetiformis. It is also used in an unlicensed manner for many dermatological conditions such as linear IgA disease, subcorneal pustular dermatosis and mucous membrane pemphigoid.

Mechanism of action

The exact mechanism by which dapsone is beneficial in inflammatory dermatoses is unknown but dapsone inhibits neutrophil chemotaxis by a number of postulated mechanisms including inhibition of both neutrophil myeloperoxidase and the adhesion of neutrophils to endothelial walls.

Formulations, doses and duration

Dapsone is only available in the United Kingdom in tablet formulation. This can present a problem in children where much smaller doses are required resulting in the unsatisfactory practice of halving and quartering tablets. In adults, the usual starting dose is 100 mg/day. This can be increased to a maximum of 200 mg to 300 mg/day although side effects become troublesome above 150 mg/day. Many patients can be maintained on much lower doses; for example, patients with dermatitis herpetiformis may only need 50 mg once or twice a week to control their disease. Duration of dosage is related to clinical course.

Monitoring and side effects

Adverse reactions to dapsone include haemolysis, neuropathy, rashes, depression and agranulocytosis. Dapsone may also cause male infertility although this is reversible.

Patients with G6PD deficiency are particularly prone to haemolysis and this enzyme should be estimated before patients are started on dapsone. Deficiency is most common but not confined to patients with Afro-Caribbean, Middle Eastern or Asian ancestry. Some degree of methaemoglobinaemia is almost invariable and may present clinically as blue lips. In situations when methaemoglobinaemia is troublesome but continued use of dapsone is desirable, some patients respond to the co-prescribing of cimetidine 400 mg tds.

Generally, full blood count and liver function tests should be estimated at baseline and regularly during dapsone therapy.

Sulfapyridine and sulfamethoxypyridazine

These drugs can be used in a similar manner to dapsone. They are available only on a named patient basis. Some practitioners prefer to use sulfamethoxypyridazine as a first line agent in the elderly because of the side effect profile of dapsone, especially depression. This is probably less common with sulfamethoxypyridazine. The dose of these drugs is usually 500 mg 2 or 3 times a day.

Antimalarials

The three antimalarials used in UK dermatological practice are chloroquine, hydroxychloroquine and mepacrine. Their most important use is in the treatment of lupus erythematosus but they can also sometimes be of help in other conditions such as porphyria cutanea tarda, dermatomyositis and sarcoidosis.

Mechanism of action

Antimalarials modify dermatological diseases by a mechanism which is as yet ill defined. Elements that may be contributory include filtering of light, immunosuppression and actions which reduce inflammation.

Formulation, doses and duration

Antimalarials are routinely given orally. An intravenous formulation of chloroquine sulphate exists but this is usually only used in serious cases of malaria. The dose of hydroxychloroquine is between 200 mg and 400 mg per day with a maximum of 6.5 mg/kg/day. Chloroquine is available in two different salts, phosphate and sulphate. Usual doses are 200 mg of chloroquine sulphate daily and its equivalent 250 mg of chloroquine phosphate daily. The upper limit of safe dosage is 4.0 mg/kg/day of chloroquine phosphate. Mepacrine is usually effective at 100 mg per day but this can be increased to 200 mg per day if required and if side effects are tolerated. All of the antimalarials usually require 6 to 8 weeks to take effect and the duration of treatment is dependent on the clinical course. Many patients with purely cutaneous lupus erythematosus require antimalarial therapy only through the summer months and are able to stop it during the winter.

The dose of chloroquine in the treatment of porphyria cutanea tarda is usually 200 mg of chloroquine sulphate twice weekly.

Monitoring and side effects

The most common adverse reaction in clinical practice is that of gastrointestinal upset. This is usually immediately apparent and while occasionally re-introduction can be successful it is common for the patient to be unable to take antimalarials in the future. The side effect that causes greatest concern is that of potential ocular toxicity. This is preventable by careful adherence to dosage and cumulative exposure. Recommendations for monitoring are available from the Royal College of Ophthalmologists website or the British National Formulary. In summary, patients without visual impairment in whom hydroxychloroquine therapy is planned can be simply screened in the dermatology clinic. Patients with visual impairment and those in whom chloroquine therapy is planned should be monitored by ophthalmologists.

Antimalarials may induce severe flares in patients with psoriasis and should therefore generally be avoided.

Mepacrine produces yellow discoloration of the skin which is often the limiting factor in its use.

Interactions

There is an increased risk of ventricular dysrhythmias when chloroquine or hydroxychloroquine is given with amiodarone or moxifloxacin. The co-prescribing of chloroquine and hydroxychloroquine with anti-epileptics may increase the risk of convulsions. The serum levels of cardiac glycosides and ciclosporin can also be increased by the co-prescribing of chloroquine and hydroxychloroquine. The absorption of chloroquine and hydroxychloroquine are reduced by the administration of kaolin and magnesium trisilicate.

Use in children

Until approximately 20 years ago the use of antimalarials was discouraged in children. They are now used judiciously in such conditions as lupus erythematosus, arthritis and dermatomyositis.

Thalidomide

Thalidomide has a notorious past history and is now subject to severe prescribing restrictions. Nevertheless, in appropriate patients it can be a very valuable and effective treatment in conditions such as lupus erythematosus, actinic prurigo, aphthous ulcers, Behçet's syndrome and nodular prurigo.

Mechanism of action

Perhaps the most interesting aspect is that the mechanism for production of teratogenicity is unknown. Thalidomide is sedating, anti-inflammatory and has effects on nervous and vascular tissue. Some of these may be as a result of modification of the action and release of TNF-α.

Formulations, doses and duration

The usual dose of thalidomide is 100 mg at night. This can be increased as far as 300 mg once daily but the sedating effect of this dose is very great indeed. Once a response is seen with thalidomide the dose can often be titrated down to as little as 50 mg three or four times a week. The duration of treatment is governed clinically but because of its potential adverse effects the drug should be given for the minimum time necessary.

Monitoring and side effects

Phocomelia with the characteristic under-developed limbs is the most common teratogenic effect of thalidomide. The peak time of susceptibility is between days 21 and 36 of pregnancy. In the United Kingdom, the main supplier of thalidomide has introduced an elaborate pregnancy prevention programme.

While teratogenicity is the most well known adverse reaction, reversible and irreversible peripheral neuropathy can also be a problem. As well as clinical monitoring, regular electrophysiological studies are recommended along with minimalization of the dose. Below 50 mg on alternate days the risk is low.

Colchicine

Colchicine is occasionally used in such conditions as Behçet's syndrome, leukocytoclastic vasculitis and palmoplantar pustulosis.

Mechanism of action

Colchicine is both anti-mitotic and anti-inflammatory. It decreases polymorphonuclear leucocyte motility and chemotaxis.

Formulations, doses and duration

Colchicine is only available orally and is given in a dose of 500 micrograms once to three times daily. The duration is dependent upon the clinical situation.

Monitoring and side effects

Many patients suffer gastrointestinal upset with colchicine, the effect being dose dependent. One interesting but rare side effect is that of myopathy. If prolonged treatment is envisaged then full blood counts should be monitored.

Interactions

Colchicine increases the plasma concentration of ciclosporin.

Intravenous immunoglobulins

Intravenous immunoglobulin is produced from pooled serum, each batch requiring approximately 10 000–15 000 donors. Elaborate measures are now undertaken to try and ensure the safety of the product. Intravenous immunoglobulin tends to be used when multiple conventional treatments have been ineffective although it is becoming a treatment of choice in a number of conditions such as Kawasaki disease, dermatomyositis and toxic epidermal necrolysis.

Mechanisms of action

There are many mechanisms which may be important in intravenous immunoglobulin therapy. These include preventing complement mediated damage, reducing pathogens and antibodies in the circulation and blockade of Fc receptors. There may also be actions due to substances within the preparation other than the antibody.

Formulations, doses and duration

Intravenous immunoglobulin is usually given at a dose of 2 grams/kg/month. This is frequently split into five consecutive doses of 0.4 grams/kg/day given by intravenous infusion. There is no agreement on how often this dose should be given but a reasonable suggestion is monthly until remission with a greater interval thereafter. Each case needs to be decided on its own merits given that the preparation is often used in conjunction with other immunosuppressants such as systemic corticosteroids and mycophenolate mofetil.

Monitoring and side effects

Intravenous immunoglobulins should be avoided in patients with isolated IgA deficiency as in these circumstances anaphylaxis can occur. It should also be avoided in patients with rapidly progressive renal disease and high titre rheumatoid factor. It is sensible to undertake a full blood count, urea and electrolytes, liver function tests, hepatitis screen, immunoglobulin levels and rheumatoid factor before starting treatment. Adverse effects are relatively rare and usually self-limiting. They can include flu-like symptoms during the infusion accompanied by tachycardia and wheezing.

Cyclophosphamide

Cyclophosphamide can be helpful in resistant cases of vasculitis and bullous disorders. It is used more frequently in haematological malignancies and rheumatological disease. Cyclophosphamide therapy has a very significant potential for acute severe side effects. It is suggested that cyclophosphamide treatment, particularly intravenous, should always be given in consultation with haematological and/or rheumatological colleagues ideally using an agreed protocol.

Mechanism of action

Cyclophosphamide is metabolized in vivo to active metabolites which produce an immunosuppressive, cytotoxic and bone marrow suppressive action. Cyclophosphamide suppresses B cells more than T cells.

Formulations, doses and duration

Cyclophosphamide is available both orally and intravenously. Oral cyclophosphamide doses range from 1 mg to 1.5 mg/kg/day. It is not necessary to induce myelosuppression to achieve immunosuppression. Cyclophosphamide can also be given as an IV pulse of 0.5 mg to 1 gram. This may be administered fortnightly or monthly often in combination with pulsed methylprednisolone. The dose and time intervals should be adjusted if renal impairment or haematological toxicity occurs.

Monitoring and side effects

Full blood count, urea and electrolytes, creatinine and liver function tests should be measured prior to treatment. Adjustments to the dose will be required if there is renal impairment. The total white cell count should be normal before instigating therapy and monitoring should take place with an expectation of lowest white cell counts 8–12 days after cyclophosphamide therapy is started.

Haemorrhagic cystitis is a significant problem in the use of cyclophosphamide and may occur in up to half of patients. To try to minimize the incidence of this it is important that patients are well hydrated during cyclophosphamide therapy. In patients receiving IV cyclophosphamide or in those who suffered haemorrhagic cystitis on previous exposure to cyclophosphamide it is recommended that mesna, which prevents toxicity by reacting with a metabolite of cyclophosphamide, should be given routinely in doses according to product literature.

Biological therapies

A new group of 'biological' therapies has been licensed in the United Kingdom for the treatment of psoriasis. These are the anti-tumour necrosis factor drugs infliximab and etanercept and the anti-leucocyte function-associated antigen-1 agent, efalizumab. They are destined to become a useful intervention for patients particularly with very severe psoriasis unresponsive to other treatments. Their main drawback is cost which is likely to severely restrict their use. They are, however, relatively less toxic than other systemic agents and are therefore attractive for both patient and doctor.

Full guidelines have been produced by the British Association of Dermatologists: the main points are summarized below.

- In order for a patient to be eligible for treatment the patient must have severe disease. For this purpose, this is defined as a Psoriasis Area and Severity (PASI) score of 10 or more (or Body Surface Area (BSA) involvement of 10% or more) and a Dermatology Life Quality Index (DLQI) score of more than 10. In addition there must be at least one other reason, for example lack of response to standard therapy or disease that is only controlled by repeated inpatient management.
- Etanercept, infliximab and efalizumab are all effective in chronic plaque psoriasis. Infliximab is also of value in unstable disease and generalized pustular psoriasis.
- Tuberculosis may be re-activated after treatment with anti-TNF agents such as infliximab. Contraindications to anti-TNF agents such as infliximab or etanercept include severe congestive heart failure or a history of demyelinating disease or optic neuritis.
- Etanercept is given by subcutaneous injection either 25 mg twice weekly or 50 mg twice weekly; intermittent courses of 24 weeks maximum are recommended. Infliximab is given over 2 hours by intravenous infusion. There is an initial induction course of 5 mg/kg at weeks 0, 2 and 6 and there are repeat infusions at 8–12 week intervals. Efalizumab is given as a subcutaneous injection, initially at a dose of 0.7 mg/kg and then as 1 mg/kg for 12 weeks: if there is a good response treatment may be continued.

Further reading

Smith CH, Anstey AV, Barker JNWN, et al. British Association of Dermatologists guidelines for use of biological intervention in psoriasis 2005. Br J Dermatol 2005; 153:486–497.

Further information

British National Formulary. Published by British Medical Association and Royal Pharmaceutical Society of Great Britain twice a year. Online. Available: www.bnf.org

British National Formulary for Children. Published by British Medical Association, Royal Pharmaceutical Society of Great Britain, Royal College of Paediatricians and Child Health and the Neonatal and Paediatric Pharmacists Group. London: 2006. New editions planned annually. Online. Available: www.bnfc.org

Electronic Medicines Compendium. Online. Available: www.emc.medicines.org.uk

Martindale: the complete drug reference. 35th edn. Sweetman SC, ed. London: Pharmaceutical Press; 2006.

Royal College of Ophthalmologists' guidelines for the monitoring of antimalarials. Online. Available: www.rcophth.ac.uk/scientific/docs/Oculartoxicity2004.pdf

British Association of Dermatologists. Online. Available: www.bad.org

Royal College Physicians of London. Corticosteroid-induced osteoporosis guidelines. Online. Available: www.rcplondon.ac.uk/pubs/books/glucocorticoid/index.asp

American Academy of Dermatology. Online. Available: www.aad.org

Prescribing unlicensed drugs or using drugs for unlicensed indications. Drugs and Therapeutics Bulletin 1992; 30(25):97–99.

Infectious diseases and infestation of the skin

8

Cherng Jong and Colin C. Long

INTRODUCTION

Skin infections and infestations are a common reason for dermatological referrals by General Practitioners (GPs) who see a large number of patients with such complaints. When skin infections or infestations become difficult to manage and chronic, they may then be referred for a dermatology opinion. Inter-departmental referral to dermatology is also common and sometimes clues of a diagnosis may be obtained by knowing the source of the referrals, e.g. cellulitis in a patient with contaminated post-operative wound. Where infection or skin infestation is suspected, it is important to take a good history, including history of recent contact with the index case and travel history. Most infections and skin infestations occur in short or recurrent bursts. This chapter attempts to briefly discuss some of the common conditions trainee dermatologists may encounter in their daily work.

UNDERSTANDING THE BASIC MICROBIOLOGY

Skin infection and infestations require the interaction between the host (human) and the offending organisms. Normally the skin is colonized by an array of micro-organisms which exist in equilibrium. For example, the forearms and back are mainly colonized by Gram-positive bacteria and yeast, whereas in the more moist groin and axilla, the organisms are more varied and numerous and include Gram-negative bacteria (Table 8.1). Skin flora can change as a result of an alteration in the local environment following the use of topical or systemic antibiotics and corticosteroids.

The skin fights foreign invasion by its physical barrier, by its normal flora providing competition to pathogenic micro-organisms and by acting as a source of fatty acids, which are toxic to many bacteria. Skin infection and signs of disease develop via three mechanisms: breach of intact skin, bloodborne infection and toxin mediated damage (Figure 8.1).

MICROBIOLOGICAL INVESTIGATIONS

It is useful to have an understanding of the basic microbiological investigation techniques in case a clinical diagnosis is not possible. These are shown in Table 8.2.

SKIN INFECTION AND INFESTATION IN A CHILD

Unlike adults, children may not be able to communicate verbally that they are unwell and therefore it is important to obtain as much information from their parents as possible about their problems. The majority of children seen in the outpatient departments are well and are also more likely to present with localized skin infection or manifestation.

Please note that some infections are described in the adult section below. Further information can be found on the British Association of Dermatologists (BAD) website

Table 8.1: The normal flora	
Body sites	**Organisms**
All body sites	*Staphylococcus aureus* *Staphylococcus epidermidis* *Micrococcus* spp.
Intertriginous areas (axilla, groin, perineum, skin folds, digital webs)	*Corynebacterium* spp. *Acinetobacter* spp. *Candida* spp.
Skin rich in sebaceous glands and hair follicles (scalp, upper back)	*Propionibacterium* spp. *Pityrosporum (Malassezia)* spp.

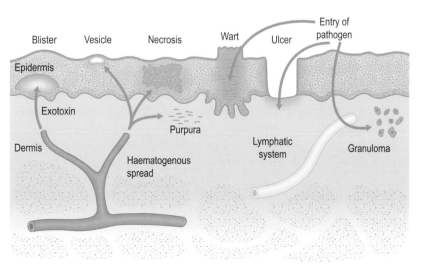

Figure 8.1
Mechanisms of mucocutaneous lesions. Invasion can occur directly via skin or from a haematogenous source. Toxins and immune complexes arrive via the latter route.

Table 8.2: *Techniques of microbiological investigations*

Techniques	Where they are indicated
Culture and sensitivity	
Skin swab	Bacterial infection
Blister fluid	Viral infection
Skin scraping	Fungal infection
Tissue biopsy	Mycobacterial infection
Staining	Bacterial infection (e.g. Gram stain)
	Mycobacterial infection (e.g. Ziehl–Neelsen for *Mycobacterium tuberculosis*)
Serum for initial and convalescence serology	Suspected viral infection
Electron microscopy	Orf
Tissue for histology	Viral infection (e.g. vacuolation, inclusion body)
Polymerase chain reaction	Viral infection, mycobacterial infection

(www.bad.org.uk) and DermNet NZ (www.dermnetnz.org). The Patient Information Leaflet section on the BAD website is a useful resource.

In a well child

Warty lesions (Figure 8.2)

Common viral warts (human papilloma virus; most commonly type 1, 2 and 4) usually present on children's fingers and as plantar warts on children's feet. These are areas exposed to repeated trauma. Warts may have areas of typical thrombosed capillaries. Asymptomatic warts do not require treatment as they will resolve spontaneously. Finger biting and sharing of personal items, for example sandals, should be discouraged. When treatment is required in painful nail fold or plantar warts, salicylic acid-based wart preparations can be used. Cryotherapy is painful and is not usually tolerated by children. For genital warts in children, the possibility of sexual abuse should be considered if there is other supporting evidence. For in-depth discussion, please refer to the BAD Guidelines.[1]

Umbilicated papular lesions (Figure 8.3)

Firm, umbilicated and sometimes scaly lesions, which appear in groups, are molluscum contagiosum caused by a poxvirus. They are usually distributed on the neck, trunk and axilla and are often asymptomatic. However, secondary bacterial infection may complicate the matter. Molluscum contagiosum may also be found in children with atopic eczema. Simple expression of lesions hastens their resolution. Sharing of personal items, e.g. towels, should be discouraged.

Crusted lesions (Figure 8.4)

Lesions with yellow or golden crust on the face and around the nose and mouth suggest impetigo (caused by *Staphylococcus* or *Streptococcus* spp.), which is much more

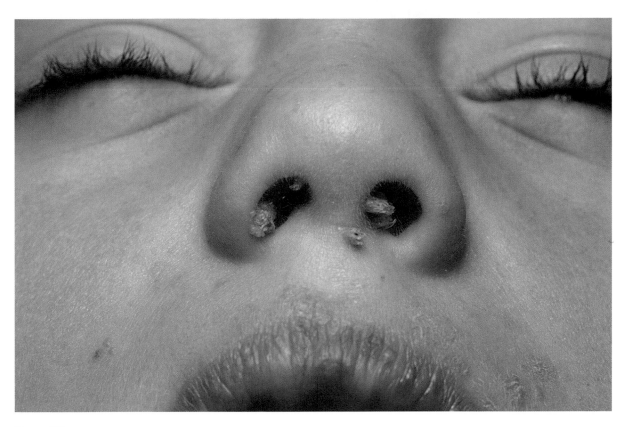

Figure 8.2
Common warts on a child's nose.

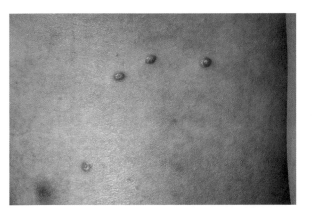

Figure 8.3
Molluscum contagiosum on a child's trunk.

commonly seen in general practice. Children who present early may have intact pustules or blisters. Impetigo is highly infectious and children often self inoculate themselves by scratching. A swab should be taken from the affected areas for bacterial culture and sensitivity if the infection recurs frequently and is slow to resolve. Treatment is with fucidin or mupirocin cream or ointment. Eradication of nasal carriage with topical mupirocin is appropriate in recurrent cases. Oral flucloxacillin, erythromycin or cephalexin may be required to treat extensive infection.

135

Grouped vesicles and erosions (Figure 8.5)

Herpes

Painful and localized vesicles, pustules or erosions suggest herpes simplex (caused by human herpesvirus 1 or 2). When the infection is localized, the child is usually asymptomatic. However, he or she may be ill with fever and enlarged regional lymph nodes. The infection is usually localized (herpes gingivostomatitis, herpes keratoconjunctivitis and herpes labialis) but in neonates it may be truncal and extensive. Referral to other specialties may be required if other organs are threatened (e.g. the eyes and genitals). For mild, localized

Figure 8.4
Staphylococcal impetigo affecting the face of a young child.

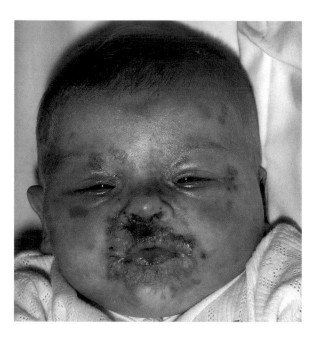

Figure 8.5
Herpes simplex affecting the periocular region.

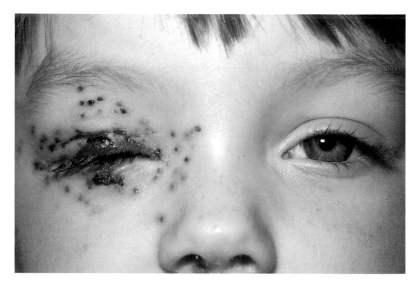

and uncomplicated herpes simplex, topical aciclovir is adequate. For severe and recurrent eruptions, treatment with oral aciclovir for short and long term (400 mg twice daily for 6 months if over 2 years of age) should be considered. The differential diagnoses of herpes zoster, impetigo and non-infective dermatosis, e.g. dermatitis herpetiformis, should be considered. Eczema herpeticum is widespread infection with herpes simplex in a patient with atopic eczema and is often misdiagnosed as bacterial infection or exacerbation of eczema. Multiple discrete crusted or vesicular lesions are seen, often affecting the face.

Hand, foot and mouth disease

In hand, foot and mouth disease (caused by coxsackie A and other enteroviruses) the vesicles are oval and they are distributed in the mouth, hands and feet of the child. These vesicles quickly break down to form ulcers that heal over a week. Viral samples taken from vesicular fluid or a throat swab can be cultured or virus can be detected by using the polymerase chain reaction (PCR) technique.

Blisters

These may be caused by insect bites, trauma (friction or thermal burns) or infection (impetigo).

A few red, scaly and annular lesions

Dermatophyte fungal infection (tinea)

Itchy, scaly, well-circumscribed and annular lesions with central clearing are suggestive of dermatophyte fungal infection or tinea (usually species from the genera *Microsporum* or *Trichophyton*). In the centre of the lesions, pustules may be occasionally found. Tinea can occur at any body site and clinical descriptions are given according to the sites involved. Tinea corporis describes tinea of the trunk and limbs; with tinea capitis (Figure 8.6); tinea pedis; tinea manuum affecting the scalp, foot and hand respectively. It is important to take

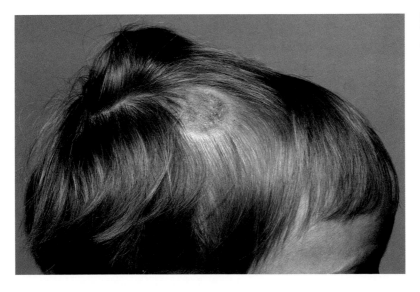

Figure 8.6
Tinea capitis on the scalp of a child.

a history to find out about the affected child's contact with pets as this may suggest a source of infection (e.g. *Microsporum canis* from dogs and cats; *Trichophyton mentagrophytes* from rodents) (Table 8.3). If tinea capitis is not treated early it may result in scarring alopecia. Kerion (Figure 8.7) is an inflamed, boggy and pustular scalp lesion usually caused by cattle ringworm.

The differential diagnoses of a scaly and well circumscribed lesion include discoid eczema and psoriasis. Atypical and non-scaly tinea resulting from inappropriate topical steroid treatment is called tinea incognito.

Hair examination under a Wood's lamp is only useful in ectothrix dermatophyte scalp hair infection (e.g. hair will fluoresce bright green in *Microsporum canis* infection).

Skin scrapings should be taken from the edge of lesions for potassium hydroxide examination and culture prior to the start of treatment. However, it may be necessary to start treatment on clinical grounds before the result is available because a positive culture result may take up to 4 weeks to become available. In tinea capitis and kerion, hair should be plucked to include the roots (not usually painful as the hair comes away easily) for potassium hydroxide examination.

Limited tinea corporis, tinea cruris, tinea manuum and tinea pedis can be treated with topical terbinafine (a fungicidal) for 2 to 4 weeks whereas tinea capitis should be treated with oral griseofulvin for 8 to 10 weeks or terbinafine (unlicensed in children) for 4 weeks or more. There are published guidelines on the management of tinea capitis.[2]

Beefy-red central erythema with satellite pustules in the nappy (diaper) area

Cutaneous candidal infection

This description is suggestive of a cutaneous candidal infection. The differential diagnoses are irritant dermatitis and flexural eczema. Topical imidazole-based (clotrimazole)

Table 8.3: Dermatophytes and their sources	
Source	**Fungi**
Anthropophilic – human	Microsporum audouinii (Africa)
	Trichophyton mentagrophytes var. mentagrophytes & var. interdigitale
	T. rubrum
	T. tonsurans
	T. violaceum (North Africa, India, Middle East)
	T. schoenleinii
	Epidermophyton floccosum
Zoophilic – animal	M. canis (cats, dogs)
	T. verrucosum (cattle)
	T. equinum (horse)
	T. mentagrophytes var. mentagrophytes (also in rodents)
	T. erinacei (hedgehogs; Europe)
	M. gallinae (fowl)
Geophilic – soil	M. gypseum

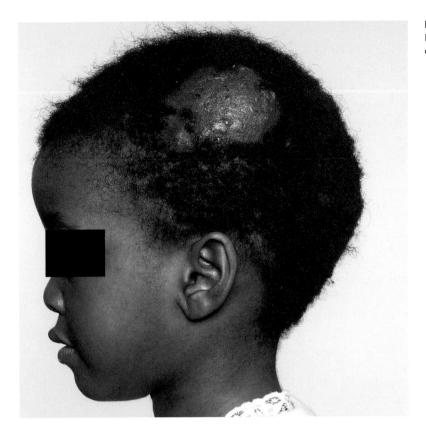

Figure 8.7
Kerion on the scalp of a child.

preparations or topical polyenes (nystatin) with each nappy change for about 5 days are effective. In cases where the diagnosis is in doubt, a skin swab for culture can be performed.

Very itchy papules on the fingers, feet and elsewhere in an irritable child

Scabies

The infant or toddler may be crying and miserable and there may be a history of contact with persons who have been treated recently with anti-scabies treatment. There are itchy papules on the interdigital webs of the fingers and flexural aspects of wrists, elbows, axillae, feet and genitalia. The papules may become excoriated in older children, as a result of intense scratching. There may be short, slightly raised, reddish brown burrows at the sites mentioned above. The GP may have tried topical steroids without any apparent benefit. The history and clinical features are very suggestive of scabies (infestation by *Sarcoptes scabiei* mite). The differential diagnosis is eczema. In crusted scabies, there is scaling of the affected areas. In doubtful cases, skin scraping taken from a burrow should be examined in a drop of potassium hydroxide or mineral oil, to look for an eight-legged mite. Treatment is by using 5% permethrin dermal cream that is applied from scalp to toe. The treatment is left on for 12 hours and then washed off. This process is repeated 7 days later to ensure good efficacy. All close contacts (persons who are in the same household) should be treated at the same time and all clothes worn within the previous week should be laundered and dried with high heat.

Head lice (Figure 8.8)

In a child with head lice, the scalp may be itchy and there may be scratch marks and excoriations. Head lice are equal opportunity parasites and they do not respect socio-economic boundaries. Infestation does not imply a lack of hygiene in their host. Head lice can be treated by using two applications of malathion, permethrin or phenothrin (leave on for 12 hours before washing off) a week apart so that all the lice that hatch within the treatment week are also treated. Encourage your patients to comb their hair with nit combs on a daily basis but not to share the combs. Choose the treatment preparations available carefully as some of them are used for short contact times only. All affected contacts and the entire household should also be treated at the same time and pillowcases and sheets should be washed and dried with high heat.

An unwell child

An unwell child is usually admitted to a paediatric ward and dermatologists may be called to see them on the ward. When there is doubt in the outpatient clinic or Accident and Emergency Department about a diagnosis or the significance of a skin sign, especially when it is extensive and when there are other systemic symptoms, the child should be admitted for observation and the management shared between the dermatology and paediatric teams.

A child with many pustules

Chickenpox

Several or numerous and widespread vesicles and pustules that appear in successive crops over a few days suggest that this is chickenpox caused by herpesvirus varicellae. The child

Figure 8.8
Head-louse eggs on hair shafts.

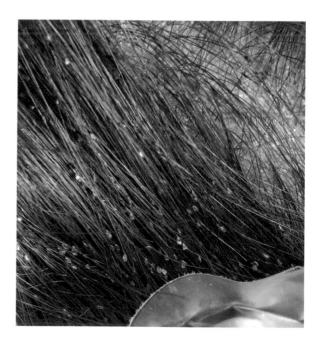

may have a low-grade fever and appear slightly unwell. The incubation period is between 2 to 3 weeks and a secondary bacterial infection of the affected skin may occur. Diagnosis is clinical and the differential diagnoses of herpes simplex and herpes zoster should be considered in patients with a more localized pustular eruption. In doubtful cases, tests can be performed (swab and culture, acute and convalescent serology, viral DNA PCR of samples taken from scraping of the base of a vesicle) after discussion with your local microbiologist. Children with mild symptoms require only symptomatic treatment, whereas in immunocompromised children oral or intravenous aciclovir are indicated. Ideally children with varicella should be isolated from other healthy individuals until all lesions have become crusted over.

When vesicles are localized to the hands, feet and mouth herpangina (caused by coxsackie A viruses) should be considered.

A child with a macular rash (Box 8.1)

Rubella

The child may have very mild symptoms or he/she may present with prodromal fever, malaise and upper respiratory symptoms. The incubation period is around 2 to 3 weeks. The child develops a macular rash that starts from the head and spreads to the toes over the next 24 hours. This rash is accompanied by occipital lymph node enlargement. The rash takes 3 days to clear. These findings are suggestive of rubella. Non-immune mothers who become exposed in the first trimester are most at risk of having an affected foetus.

Measles

Measles causes a similar but more of a maculopapular rash and it spreads from the face to involve other parts of the body more slowly, over 2 to 3 days. The prodromal symptoms in patients with measles are very similar to those that occur in rubella but in measles the incubation period is slightly longer. Preauricular lymph nodes may be enlarged and white Koplik spots may be found on the buccal mucosa. Measles may be complicated by otitis media, pneumonia and encephalitis.

An acute and a convalescence serology to detect acute immunoglobulin M and a four-fold rise in immunoglobulin G can be done to detect and confirm these infections. Active vaccination is available for both conditions and human normal immunoglobulin is indicated in immunocompromised children, non-immune pregnant women and infants under 9 months, who have been exposed to measles.

Box 8.1: *Causes of a macular rash*

- Rubella
- Measles
- Erythema infectiosum
- Roseola
- Infectious mononucleosis
- Scarlet fever
- Drug eruption

Erythema infectiosum

Erythema infectiosum (infection caused by human parvovirus B19) can also cause a macular rash. This usually starts with intense redness of the cheek (slapped-cheek appearance) and later the child develops a more widespread lacy pink or dull-red macular rash involving the trunk, arms and legs. The incubation period is between 1 to 2 weeks and the disease is transmitted via respiratory droplets or blood products. If the child appears anaemic, the full blood count should be checked, as aplastic crisis is a recognized complication. In pregnant women infected during the first and second trimesters, foetal monitoring may be indicated. Immunoglobulin M can be measured to detect an acute infection. Uncomplicated infection only requires symptomatic treatment.

Roseola

In roseola (caused by human herpesvirus 6), the child usually has a high fever and when the fever subsides, a rose pink papular eruption appears on the trunk and neck. The incubation period is about 2 weeks. The disease is transmitted by saliva or respiratory droplets. The child is usually under 3 years of age. The infection may be complicated by febrile convulsions because of the high fever. Uncomplicated infection only requires symptomatic treatment.

Infectious mononucleosis

Older children or adolescents are more likely to have infectious mononucleosis caused by Epstein–Barr virus. The incubation period is 1 to 2 months. Patients usually have a fever, lymphadenopathy and a sore throat that may have been treated recently with penicillin. Hepatosplenomegaly sometimes occurs. Splenic rupture, thrombocytopenia, haemolytic anaemia and cardiac involvement are rare but they do happen. Therefore it is important to examine all patients with rashes thoroughly. When infectious mononucleosis is suspected it is important to perform a full blood count and the diagnosis should be supported by a Paul–Bunnell test or Monospot screening test. Both these tests detect a heterophile antibody (immunoglobulin M) that agglutinates mammalian red cells. Serology to detect specific immunoglobulin M and a rising immunoglobulin G should also be performed. Anti-streptolysin O titre should be checked to exclude scarlet fever.

Scarlet fever

Scarlet fever (caused by *Streptococcus pyogenes*) is characterized by a rapid onset of fever, anorexia, tonsillitis and lymphadenopathy. An erythematous macular rash spreads from the neck downward over the trunk to the extremities. A white or red strawberry tongue, circumoral pallor and linear petechiae (along skin folds) may be found. Anti-streptolysin O titre should be performed to confirm the diagnosis. The disease can be treated with penicillin for 10 days. Possible complications from this disease are myocarditis, rheumatic fever, arthritis, osteomyelitis and meningitis.

A child with a purpuric rash

Meningococcaemia

In an unwell child this raises the concern of meningococcaemia and the patient should be managed by a paediatric team. Initial blind therapy using benzylpenicillin (child

1 month–18 years 50 mg/kg every 4–6 hours; adult 2.4 g every 4 hours) or cefotaxime (child 1 month–18 years 50 mg/kg every 8–12 hours; adult 2 g every 6 hours) should be given urgently.

A child with erythematous skin and desquamation

SSSS, TSS and TEN

There are several differential diagnoses to consider: staphylococcal scalded skin syndrome (SSSS), toxic shock syndrome (TSS) and toxic epidermal necrolysis (TEN). In SSSS, the child, usually under the age of 5 years, may have a focus of infection (e.g. skin, respiratory tract), which is followed by a fever and a widespread erythematous eruption and blister formation. The skin becomes tender to touch and gentle rubbing on the skin results in epidermal separation, leaving a shiny, moist and red surface (i.e. positive Nikolsky's sign). Periorbital and perioral crusting may be evident.

TSS, on the other hand, can occur at any age but typically in adolescents and young adults. Often, a focus of skin infection is evident. All patients have a fever and hypotension. They may have evidence of renal failure. Patients may develop a scarlatiniform rash which is followed a week or two later by desquamation of the skin on the palms and soles.

TSS may be caused by *Staphylococcus aureus* or Group A *Streptococcus* and both TSS and SSSS are mediated by an exotoxin. Blood should be taken for culture and sensitivity. TEN may be confused with SSSS and in both cases the Nikolsky sign is positive. In TEN, the dusky red skin is necrotic and it comes off in large sheets. Skin biopsy specimens show a subepidermal split in TEN, and a subcorneal split in SSSS.

The choice of antibiotics in SSSS and TSS should be discussed with the local microbiologists, e.g. beta-lactamase resistant antibiotics: flucloxacillin to cover staphylococci and co-amoxiclav to cover streptococci.

SKIN INFECTION AND INFESTATION IN AN ADULT PATIENT

- Please note some infections are described in the children's section above.

Viral warts and molluscum contagiosum

Viral warts

Although the majority of patients with viral warts seen in the outpatient department are immunocompetent, viral warts are more likely to develop and become more numerous in patients who are immunosuppressed, e.g. patients on long term immunosuppressive drugs such as tacrolimus, azathioprine, ciclosporin or who have human immunodeficiency virus (HIV) infection. Patients have usually tried topical preparations containing salicylic acid. Salicylic acid should be avoided for warts on the face as it can cause severe irritation at that site. Adults are tolerant of physical destructive treatment, e.g. cryotherapy or curettage, when there is a small number of warts.

Genital warts are treated with 5% topical imiquimod cream, three times a week for 16 weeks. Alternatively, purified podophyllotoxin 0.5% solution, which is applied twice daily for three consecutive days, can be used under the direct supervision of a treating physician. This treatment may need to be repeated to produce clinical clearance.

Molluscum contagiosum

In adults this is more commonly seen in association with atopic eczema or with immunosuppression due to HIV infection or immunosuppressant drugs. The papules can be treated by expression of their content, cryotherapy or by applying 5% imiquimod cream three times a week for 4 weeks.

Discrete inflamed pustules and tender red nodules

Pseudomonas *folliculitis, pseudofolliculitis barbae and* Malassezia furfur

Lesions arising as a result of exogenous infection are usually confined to hair bearing areas. The presentation of a pus-containing lesion depends on the depth of the lesion and it ranges from a pustule (in folliculitis) to a tender red nodule (a furuncle). The predisposing factors are: occlusive bandaging in the treatment of eczema (seen on dermatology wards), diabetes, obesity, long term antibiotic and corticosteroid use. Hot tub usage is associated with *Pseudomonas* folliculitis. A skin swab should be taken for culture and sensitivity. Flucloxacillin or a macrolide is the treatment of choice. Pustules on the beard area may be due to a foreign body reaction called pseudofolliculitis barbae. In recurrent cases this is treated with long term tetracycline and patients should be advised to reduce frequency of shaving. Folliculitis on the back may be due to *Malassezia furfur*; this is treated with miconazole cream.

Large red and hot area on a limb

Cellulitis

This is usually either cellulitis or a deep vein thrombosis or both. In cellulitis (affecting the dermis and subcutaneous tissue), the skin is erythematous and has a spreading edge and tracking proximal red streaks due to lymphangitis. Regional lymph nodes may be enlarged and there may be signs of the source of infection (e.g. fungal infection between the toes, fissured eczema or a thorn injury). The affected limb is swollen and painful and the patient may be pyrexial. A skin swab and blood culture should be taken. Erythema nodosum can appear very similar to cellulitis but erythema nodosum usually consists of several diffusely red large raised nodules. Cellulitis is treated with flucloxacillin (for staphylococci) and benzylpenicillin (for streptococci) or a macrolide such as erythromycin if the patient is allergic to penicillin, for 14 days. Dermatologists are often asked to see patients who have had several courses of antibiotics for cellulitis associated with a chronic leg ulcer. In such cases, one should always make sure that the 'cellulitis' is not contact dermatitis or redness due to haemosiderin deposition or lipodermatosclerosis.

Erysipelas

Erysipelas (Figure 8.9) is usually more clearly demarcated (affects the dermis) than cellulitis and is less swollen. It may occur on the face, legs and feet.

Necrotizing fasciitis

If there has been a rapid deterioration of an area of cellulitis including the skin turning blue-grey, bullae formation, a malodorous discharge and crepitation, the diagnosis of necrotizing fasciitis should be considered. The patient is usually ill with fever, diarrhoea, nausea and vomiting. There may be a history of recent surgery, ulcer formation or penetrating trauma affecting the lower limbs, abdomen or perineum. Surgeons should be consulted for surgical debridement of necrotic skin. Depending on the sites and suspected organisms, a broad spectrum antibiotic with Gram positive and Gram negative cover (e.g. penicillin G for Group A *Streptococcus* and *Clostridium* spp.), metronidazole (for anaerobes) and gentamicin or piperacillin/tazobactam (for *Pseudomonas* infection) may be required. Appropriate samples (skin, blood, urine, faeces) should be sent for culture and sensitivity.

An adult with grouped vesicles and erosion

Herpes infections

Herpes simplex also occurs in adults and it usually affects the perioral region and less commonly the fingers. When one or several dermatomes are involved, e.g. trigeminal or thoracic dermatoses, shingles/herpes zoster should be considered. Ophthalmology advice is required in ophthalmic zoster because this can be accompanied by zoster keratitis, and blindness if untreated. Herpes zoster is treated with intravenous aciclovir or oral valaciclovir (better oral absorption than aciclovir) or oral aciclovir, as soon as possible, to

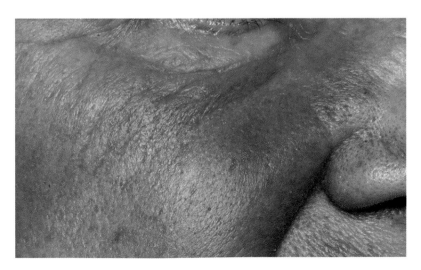

Figure 8.9
Erysipelas affecting a woman's cheek.

limit disease progression and to reduce the risk of post-herpetic neuralgia. The staff on the ward will need to know that patients with herpes zoster will require isolation until the blisters have dried up. Severe and recurrent herpes simplex cases, and especially when these are accompanied by erythema multiforme, should be treated with short and then long term (400 mg twice daily for 6 months) aciclovir respectively.

An ill adult with numerous pustules

Chickenpox

Chickenpox occurs less frequently in adults but adults tend to suffer more severe systemic symptoms. There is also a higher chance of developing complications, e.g. pneumonia and hepatitis.

A farmer who has a reddish-blue swelling on a finger

Orf

In orf (Figure 8.10), the lesion usually starts off as a small papule which develops into a haemorrhagic nodule or pustule. Often there is a central crust. The patient may have

Figure 8.10
Orf on a finger.

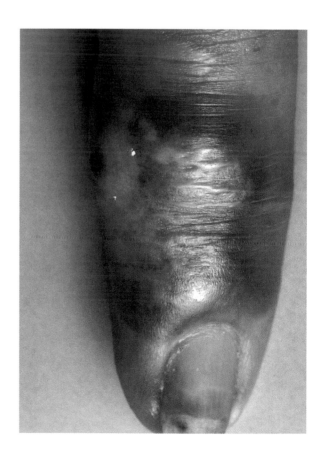

regional lymph node enlargement and fever. The parapoxvirus is acquired from handling sheep, goat, meat or from a contaminated barn door or feeding trough. The disease is usually diagnosed clinically but can be confirmed histologically and with electron microscopy.

A keeper of tropical fish with a non-healing plaque on the hand or nodules in a sporotrichoid distribution on an arm

Fish tank granuloma

The nodules, sometimes in a sporotrichoid distribution along the line of lymphatic vessels, are suggestive of fish tank granuloma (Figure 8.11) caused by *Mycobacterium marinum* infection acquired from handling fish or cleaning out a fish tank. A tissue biopsy should be obtained for culture. The infection is treated with minocycline, rifampicin or co-trimoxazole for 3 months.

Thick and crumbly nails (Figure 8.12)

Dermatophyte infection

Dermatophyte infection due to *Trichophyton rubrum* is the most common cause of nail infections. Nail clippings and scrapings should be sent for microscopy and culture. Dermatophyte infection is treated with terbinafine for 6 weeks for finger nail infection and 12 weeks for toe nail infection. Candida onychomycosis is treated with two to four pulses of itraconazole (1 week per month). There are published guidelines on the treatment of onychomycosis.[3]

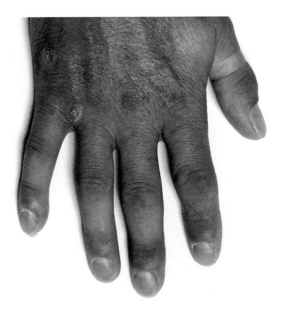

Figure 8.11
Purple-red nodules of *Mycobacterium marinum* infection.

Figure 8.12
Onychomycosis.

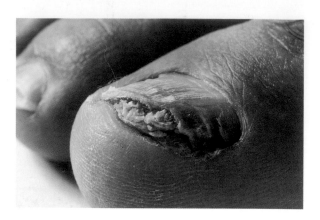

Numerous itchy papules and crusted eczema-like areas in an elderly patient

Scabies

The scenario is usually of an elderly person who has been admitted from a nursing home or a long-stay ward (e.g. elderly care or rehabilitation ward). This history is suggestive of scabies. The patient may have several itchy red papules on the fingers and the scrotum in men. Less commonly, a patient with, for example, Parkinson's disease or stroke may have crusted eczema-like areas called crusted or Norwegian scabies. The treatment is the same as in children but be prepared to see another 20 affected patients and staff on the same ward! Oral ivermectin may be indicated for crusted scabies.

Multiple white or brown pink patches with fine scaling on the trunk and upper arms

Pityriasis versicolor

Asymptomatic multiple fine-scaled hyperpigmented (pale-skinned individuals) or hypopigmented (dark-skinned individuals) patches on the trunk, axillae and limbs are suggestive of pityriasis versicolor caused by a yeast called *Malassezia furfur*. GPs or other physicians may query vitiligo in their referral letters. The other differential diagnosis is pityriasis alba which is seen (usually on the face) in atopic individuals. Where diagnosis is difficult, Wood's lamp examination (yellow fluorescence in pityriasis versicolor) and skin scraping and potassium hydroxide examination (looking for hyphae and spores) are useful. The treatment options include selenium sulfide or ketoconazole shampoo, ketoconazole cream daily for 10 days, or oral itraconazole (child 1 month–12 years: 3–5 mg/kg [maximum 200 mg] once daily for a week; child 12–18 years and adults: 200 mg once daily for a week).

Multiple coppery red papules and plaques

Syphilis

The differential diagnoses to be considered here are pityriasis rosea, lichen planus and syphilis. In syphilis the palms are usually affected and there may be associated signs of fever, weight loss and generalized lymphadenopathy, which are not seen in pityriasis rosea. Diagnosis is by non-specific screening tests using rapid plasma reagin and Venereal Disease Research Laboratory tests, and by specific tests using *Treponema pallidum* haemagglutination assay, microhaemagglutination assay for antibodies to *Treponema pallidum* or the fluorescent treponemal antibody absorption test. Syphilis is treated with procaine benzylpenicillin for 14 days.

Skin infection in a returned traveller

It is essential to enquire where the patient has travelled from and the activities that they have carried out while overseas. They may remember they have been bitten by insects.

Cutaneous larva migrans

A intensely itchy, creeping, raised, serpiginous and erythematous tract suggests cutaneous larva migrans (Figure 8.13). The organisms responsible for this condition are *Ancylostoma braziliensis*, *Necator americanus* and *Strongyloides stercoralis*, which are acquired by walking barefoot. These organisms are distributed in Europe, Asia and other tropical areas such as the West Indies. Eggs and larvae may be found in the faeces in systemic infection. Localized disease is treated with topical 10% thiabendazole (made from crushed thiabendazole tablets) whereas systemic infection is treated with a single dose of ivermectin.

Lupus vulgaris

Any brown plaque on a patient from Asia or Southern Africa should alert a dermatologist to the diagnosis of lupus vulgaris. The differential diagnosis is sarcoidosis and a biopsy sample should be taken for Ziehl–Neelsen staining and culture or polymerase chain reaction to detect mycobacterial DNA. Chest X-ray should be taken to exclude pulmonary tuberculosis. Lupus vulgaris is treated with isoniazid, rifampicin, pyrazinamide and ethambutol for the first 2 months and isoniazid and rifampicin for a further 4 months.

Leprosy

A hypopigmented patch, an anaesthetic plaque with red, raised edges or numerous hypopigmented or red macules of a patient from the Far East, Africa or South America

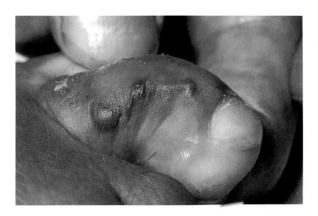

Figure 8.13
Cutaneous larva migrans affecting a patient's toe.

may suggest leprosy. A skin scraping, a swab taken of the nasal secretion or a slit skin smear should be taken for staining with Ziehl–Neelsen to look for *Mycobacterium leprae*.

Erythema chronicum migrans

A large and expanding erythematous plaque on the leg after returning from a camping trip in Europe or North America could indicate erythema chronicum migrans caused by *Borrelia burgdorferi* (Lyme disease). The patient may not recall a tick bite. Localized skin disease is treated by amoxicillin 1 g three times a day or doxycycline 100 mg twice a day for 3 weeks. Systemic infection, where there is lymphadenopathy, and complicated cases where there may be arthritis, myocarditis, neuropathies, meningoencephalitis or hepatitis, should be treated with intravenous ceftriaxone 2 g daily for 2 weeks. The infection can be confirmed by the detection of an antibody to *Borrelia burgdorferi* but this will need to be confirmed subsequently with a Western blot analysis. The positive predictive value of these serology tests depends on the local prevalence of Lyme disease (uncommon in the United Kingdom) and therefore the opinion of a microbiologist should be sought at an early stage.

Cutaneous leishmaniasis

A nodule or a non-healing ulcer that has developed over several months on the arm or nasal mucosa in a traveller from the Mediterranean basin, Northern Africa, India or South America suggests the lesion may be cutaneous leishmaniasis. A slit skin smear or a tissue biopsy should be obtained, stained and examined to look for parasites. Tissue histology may show granuloma. DNA detection using the polymerase chain reaction technique and tissue culture are available in some hospitals. The treatment of different species of *Leishmania* should be discussed with a microbiologist or infectious diseases specialist.

CONCLUSION

There are a wide number of skin infections and infestations. The diagnosis is based largely on clinical grounds but if in doubt, the case should be discussed with a consultant colleague, a consultant microbiologist or an infectious diseases consultant. Unlike idiopathic inflammatory skin diseases, most skin infections and infestations can be cured and this makes treating skin infections and infestations a very rewarding task.

References

1. Sterling JC, Handfield-Jones S, Hudson PM. Guidelines for the management of cutaneous warts. Br J Dermatol 2001; 144:4–11.
2. Higgins EM, Fuller LC, Smith CH. Guidelines for the management of tinea capitis. Br J Dermatol 2000; 143:53–58.
3. Roberts DT, Taylor WD, Boyle J. Guidelines for treatment of onychomycosis. Br J Dermatol 2003; 148:402–410.

Dressings and wound care

9

Angela Steen and Diane J. Williamson

INTRODUCTION

Chronic leg ulceration is already a common problem in Western society and is likely to become more prevalent with our ageing population. The cost of leg ulcers is enormous both in terms of morbidity and finance. This cost can be partly addressed by expeditious treatment of leg ulcers by experienced doctors and nurses in a multidisciplinary setting.

Until recently, many doctors perceived leg ulceration as a chronic, incurable problem and the management of patients with leg ulcers has been largely neglected in both undergraduate and postgraduate medical teaching. As leg ulcers do not automatically fall under one specialist category, it has been left to specialists in varying fields such as dermatology, diabetology, vascular and plastic surgery to develop subspecialist interests in the management of these patients. Traditionally, nurses have shouldered the burden of work by becoming intrinsically involved with the patient management through regular contact with patients when applying wound dressings and bandaging. Many nurses, however, still feel unsupported when complications arise due to the lack of specialist knowledge of their medical colleagues in this area. Fortunately, this situation is beginning to change and doctors are now increasingly realizing the important role which they have to play in both the direct management of these patients and in supporting their nursing colleagues.

THE COST OF LEG ULCERATION

In the UK, chronic leg ulceration is estimated to affect approximately 0.15–0.18% of the population. This extrapolates to approximately 100 000 patients who suffer with chronic leg ulceration in the UK at any one time. Most of these patients are over 65 and it is likely that as the population ages, this prevalence will increase.

Multiple studies have demonstrated a profound adverse effect of leg ulceration on quality of life. For younger patients, loss of earnings is a major consideration. Pain, restriction in physical and social functioning and perceived poorer general health have been demonstrated at all ages.

In a National Health Service which is constantly trying to control spiralling costs, the financial implications of managing leg ulceration has to be taken seriously. For chronic leg ulceration alone, without giving consideration to other wound management, the cost has been estimated in the UK as approximately £200 million per year. This cost reflects nursing time, dressing and bandage costs and medical care as well as loss of patient earnings.

In order to reduce patient morbidity and healthcare costs, dermatologists must play a major role in both the multidisciplinary management of patients with leg ulceration and in teaching and promoting good practices of wound care to other healthcare professionals.

This chapter is intended to provide a practical approach to the management of patients with leg ulceration. For detailed information on aetiopathogenesis, the reader is referred to dermatology reference books.

STAGES OF WOUND HEALING

In order for the clinician to understand chronic wounds, a basic understanding of the normal stages of wound healing is required.

Wounds should progress through four stages of healing in a timely and orderly fashion. Much of the research in chronic wound healing is currently focused on factors influencing progression through these stages. This research may help some chronic wounds, which appear to get 'stuck' in a certain stage.

1. Haemostasis — tissue injury provokes immediate activation of the coagulation pathways resulting in fibrin formation. This acts as a temporary plug to close the wound.
2. Inflammation — neutrophils initially clear the wound of debris which may impair wound healing. Macrophages release cytokines which provide the correct environment for promotion of new tissue formation. Additionally, they produce extracellular molecules which combine with others to produce a provisional matrix which serves as a scaffold for dermal regeneration and epidermal migration and proliferation.
3. Proliferation — angiogenesis provides capillary loops within the provisional matrix which gives the wound its red granular appearance — hence the term granulation tissue. Fibroblasts proliferate and migrate into the provisional matrix and synthesize collagen. Epithelial cell proliferation and migration then occurs.
4. Remodelling — this transitory phase from granulation tissue to scar involves reorganization and maturation of collagen fibres. During this phase, the wound is converted from approximately 20% normal, unwounded tensile strength to approximately 70–80% strength of normal skin. This process can last for up to 1–2 years after the wound has appeared to heal externally.

ASSESSMENT OF LEG ULCERS

Most of the causes of leg ulceration together with co-factors which can impair healing are listed in Table 9.1. As ulcers are more common in the elderly, it is not uncommon to have

Table 9.1: Aetiological factors and co-factors in leg ulceration

Causes of leg ulceration	Co-factors which impair healing
Venous insufficiency and dependency (70%)	Anaemia
Arterial occlusion (10%)	Old age
Diabetic (10%)	Infection
Other (10%)	Malnutrition
Pressure (decubitus)	Immunosuppressants/chemotherapeutic agents
Pyoderma gangrenosum	NSAIDs
Vasculitic ulceration	Psychosocial stress
Malignancy	
Sickle cell disease	
Hydroxyurea-induced	
Hypertensive ulcer	
Dermatitis artefacta	
Infection	
Microcirculatory disorders	
Neuropathic diseases	
Clotting disorders	
Metabolic diseases	

multi-aetiological ulcers with numerous co-factors present. Although the vast majority of leg ulcers in the community are primarily venous in origin, the aetiology of those presenting to outpatient dermatology clinics also includes the more complex vasculitic, rheumatoid, pyoderma gangrenosum and multi-aetiological ulcers. The other conditions mentioned in Table 9.1 are rare and should be considered when an ulcer cannot be categorized into one or more of the more common causes, when the ulcer fails to respond to treatment or in case of additional clinical signs or laboratory abnormalities.

Before considering what dressings to use in the management of leg ulceration, the cause(s) and any important co-factors which are thought to be delaying healing must be elicited and addressed. This requires a full assessment of the patient in the form of history, examination and investigation as appropriate (Table 9.4).

History and examination

In view of the often multi-aetiological nature of leg ulcers, a full history (Box 9.1) and examination are essential. If pyoderma gangrenosum is suspected, care should be taken to elicit the exact way in which the ulcer started, in which case a history of pathergy or pustule formation can be extremely helpful.

History and examination must include vascular assessment, as arteriosclerosis is common in the elderly and may be a co-factor if not a direct aetiological factor. It is helpful to measure the length and width of ulcers to allow progress to be monitored objectively. This is done by measuring the longest ulcer length and the longest perpendicular width (Figure 9.1).

153

Box 9.1: *Clinical notes: history taking in leg ulceration*

General

- Occupation, e.g. standing all day
- Date ulcer started
- How ulcer started
- History of previous leg ulcers
- Ulcer pain
- Type and severity of pain
- Impact of leg ulcers on life

Indicators of venous disease

- Varicose veins
- Surgery for varicose veins
- Deep venous thrombosis
- Fracture in affected limb
- Joint surgery
- Major surgery
- Number of pregnancies

Indicators of arterial disease

- Hypertension
- CVA/TIA
- Ischaemic heart disease/MI
- Intermittent claudication
- Rest pain
- Diabetes mellitus — including duration
- Smoking history

Other

- Rheumatoid arthritis
- Obesity
- Anaemia
- Mobility, e.g. unrestricted, walks to garden, walks around house, immobile
- Medication

Figure 9.1
Ulcer healing can be monitored by measuring length and width as shown.

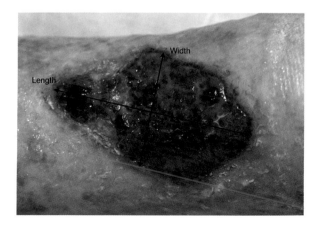

Handheld Doppler examination

In combination with a complete clinical assessment, Doppler ultrasound (Figure 9.2a, b and c) is used to confirm the presence or absence of arterial disease (Box 9.2).

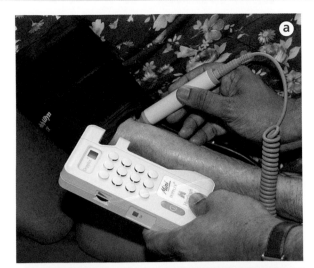

Figure 9.2
(a, b and c) Handheld Doppler ultrasound examination.

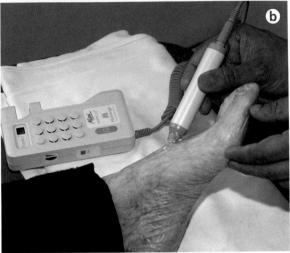

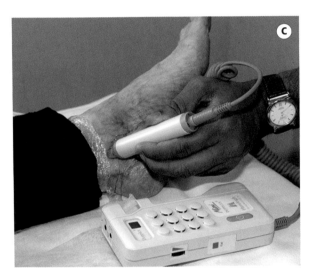

Box 9.2: Procedure for recording Doppler Ankle Brachial Pressure Index (ABPI)

1. Lie patient supine for 10–20 minutes (to negate effects of exercise on BP) and explain procedure
2. Apply protection over any ulcers, e.g. with cling film
3. Apply correct size of cuff around upper arm
4. Locate brachial pulse and apply ultrasound gel
5. Angle the Doppler probe at 45–60 degrees and locate pulse
6. Inflate cuff until audible sound disappears
7. Release cuff slowly and record pressure at which signal reappears
8. Repeat the procedure using the other arm. Use the higher of the two brachial pressure measurements to calculate ABPI
9. Apply appropriate size cuff to ankle immediately above the malleolus
10. Locate dorsalis pedis by palpation and apply ultrasound gel and probe as before
11. Inflate and deflate cuff as previously and record when signal reappears
12. Locate posterior tibial pulse and repeat procedure. Take the higher of the latter two readings to calculate ABPI
13. Perform the same procedure on the other leg
14. To calculate the ABPI divide the higher ankle pressure for each leg by the higher brachial pressure obtained

$$\frac{\text{Highest ankle pressure}}{\text{Highest brachial pressure}} = \text{Ankle Brachial Pressure Index (ABPI)}.$$

A crystal in the Doppler probe transmits sound waves, which are reflected back by moving red blood cells. These are received by a second crystal and transmitted into audible sounds.

An ankle brachial pressure index (ABPI) of 0.9–1.0 is considered normal. In general, indices below 0.8 signify some arterial disease. More severe clinical symptoms such as rest pain are usually found with ABPI of < 0.5, while readings between 0.5 and 0.8 may be associated with intermittent claudication.

ABPI of > 1.0 should be interpreted with caution as this may suggest calcification of vessels (see below). Further investigation may be required in these patients to assess the degree of arterial disease.

Pitfalls with handheld Doppler examination

There are certain clinical scenarios in which Doppler readings can be misleading, potentially resulting in inappropriate management with disastrous clinical outcomes (Box 9.3). Doppler results must therefore always be interpreted together with the clinical assessment and should be used to confirm clinical findings. A reading which is discordant with clinical findings should be considered aberrant until otherwise proven.

Box 9.3: Advantages and disadvantages of handheld Doppler

Advantages

- Non-invasive
- Easily performed
- Outpatient procedure

Disadvantages

- In approximately 10% of the elderly population and in patients with diabetes, calcification of the medial layer of the distal arteries occurs, rendering them incompressible and yields a falsely elevated ankle brachial pressure index (ABPI)
- Gross oedema can confound ABPI results
- Inter-observer variability demonstrated in some studies
- Lack of reproducibility demonstrated in some studies

Doppler waveforms

With more sophisticated machines, but using the same technique, a graphic waveform may also be produced that can be used as an adjunct to overall vascular assessment (Figure 9.3a, b and c). This is particularly helpful for those patients in whom ABPI is artificially elevated due to the calcification of the vessels. A normal waveform is triphasic. If mild arterial disease exists proximal to the probe, waveforms become biphasic, with monophasic waveforms in the presence of more severe disease.

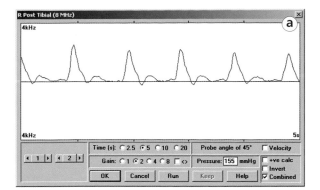

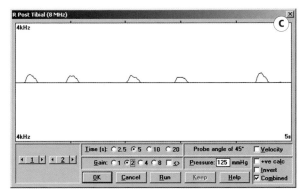

Figure 9.3
(a) Triphasic waveforms. (b) Biphasic waveforms.
(c) Monophasic waveforms.

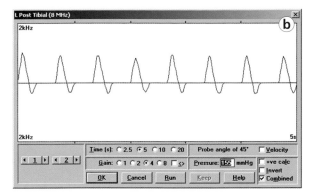

Pulse oximetry

Pulse oximetry can also be used as an alternative to Doppler examination with some advantages over Doppler. It is more reliable than Doppler examination in patients with significant oedema and is a simple, easily maintained skill. The pulse oximetry sensor is applied to a digit and a blood pressure cuff is applied as for a normal Doppler. The cuff is inflated and deflated and the pressure is recorded at which the pulse oximetry signal is lost. The toe/finger oximetry index is similar to the Doppler ABPI, such that it is safe to apply high compression therapy with a toe/finger index of > 0.8. If there is any doubt, compression bandaging can be applied and the signal checked with the leg horizontal and elevated. Loss of signal or a significant drop in SpO_2 (oxyhaemoglobin saturation) indicates that further assessment is necessary before proceeding with compression.

Duplex ultrasonography

In some patients, further investigations may help to elucidate the degree of arterial disease. Duplex ultrasonography can provide non-invasive, accurate information regarding site and nature of vascular lesions. Its sensitivity is greatest above the knee where it has comparable diagnostic capabilities to angiography in the assessment of arterial occlusive disease in patients with symptoms of peripheral vascular disease.

VENOUS LEG ULCERS

Typically, patients with venous leg ulcers have a history of either deep venous thrombosis or varicose veins, or predisposing factors for these, such as multiple pregnancies, major abdominal operations or fractured limbs.

Venous leg ulceration can occur anywhere within the gaiter area of the leg, although it is much more common over the malleolar area. Most venous leg ulcers occur over the medial malleolus where there are a high proportion of perforator veins, which transmit the high pressure to the superficial venous system.

Clinical signs of venous hypertension seen in the gaiter area of the leg
(Figure 9.4)

- Peripheral oedema
- Varicose veins
- Venous flare
- Hyperpigmentation
- Atrophie blanche
- Leg ulceration
- Venous eczema
- Lipodermatosclerosis

Management involves demonstration of venous incompetence, either clinically or by investigations such as venous duplex scan. Once venous incompetence has been established, graduated compression of the affected leg is the treatment of choice, *providing clinical and Doppler examination has excluded significant arterial disease.*

Figure 9.4
Varicosities and
hyperpigmentation in a
patient with venous
hypertension

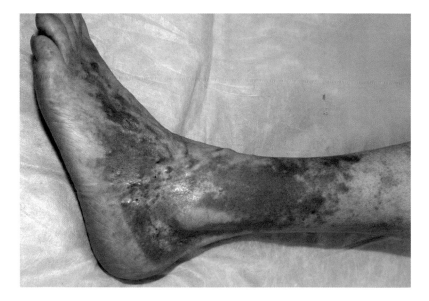

COMPRESSION THERAPY

Below knee, graduated, high compression in the form of bandages or hosiery is the main treatment in the management of uncomplicated venous leg ulcers. Treatment reduces pain and oedema, and enhances quality of life through improved healing rates. High, multi-layer compression has been shown to be more effective than low or single layer compression. Inappropriate application of compression in the presence of arterial disease can result in reduction in blood flow, which can potentially lead to gangrene.

Prior to application of compression, a full vascular examination should be performed. This should include an arterial Doppler examination; however, this should not be taken in isolation. The Doppler result should be used to confirm the findings from your clinical examination.

When is it safe to apply compression?

There is currently no evidence to indicate at what level high compression may be safely applied to a limb; however, current opinion states that high compression should not be applied to a limb with an ABPI of < 0.8. Modified or low compression may be used by experienced clinicians in patients with ABPI 0.6–0.8.

How can graduated compression be applied?

According to Laplace's law, the sub-bandage pressure applied is directly related to both tension in the bandage and limb circumference (Box 9.4). Therefore, in a normal shaped limb, a bandage applied with constant tension and overlap will achieve graduated compression with the greater compression at the ankle. Recommended high compression is 40 mmHg at the ankle reducing to 15–20 mmHg at the calf.

Box 9.4: Laplace's law

Sub-bandage pressure = (tension) × (no. of layers) × (constant)/(circumference of limb) × (bandage width)

Which bandage should I use? (Figure 9.5)

There are many different bandage systems available, each with different properties. No studies have shown superiority of one specific bandage system over another. In general, high compression is better than low compression for the treatment of venous leg ulcers. Patient concerns such as bandage bulkiness, comfort and lifestyle should therefore be considered when applying compression bandaging to aid concordance.

Elastic bandages (e.g. Setopress®)

- Also known as long stretch or highly extensible bandage.
- Produces sustained compression with high pressure at rest. When the calf muscles expand during walking, the bandage expands producing slightly less but still high pressure.
- Able to accommodate changes in limb circumference when oedema reduced, i.e. bandages still effective when oedema has reduced.

Figure 9.5
A selection of currently available compression bandages.

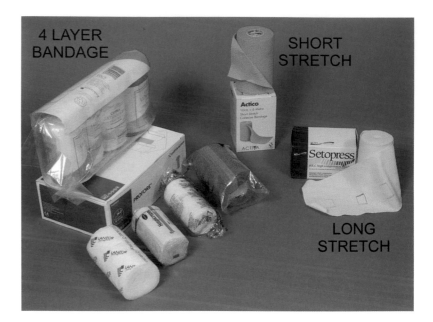

Inelastic bandages (e.g. Comprilan®)

- Also known as short stretch bandage.
- Provides a relatively rigid system which produces high compression during walking (when calf muscle contracts against the fixed bandage) but low resting pressures.
- Unable to conform to accommodate any reduction in oedema. This may result in bandages falling down if not changed more frequently during initial application.

Multi-layer bandage systems (e.g. Profore™)

- Three or four layers including padding and crêpe and a variety of inelastic/elastic and cohesive bandages.
- Can be bulky leading to difficulty with footwear.
- Various systems are available that combine advantages of both compression systems.

ARTERIAL LEG ULCERATION

Arterial ulceration usually presents as painful, punched out ulcers on the dorsum of the foot, or distal gangrene affecting the toes. A significant number of patients, however, present with ulcers on the lower leg, often precipitated by trauma, which have a predominant arterial element. Again, these are usually painful and patients typically have a history of intermittent claudication with or without rest pain. Peripheral pulses are diminished or absent and the limb is often cold and dusky with delayed capillary refill time. Exposed tendon may be visible in the base of the ulcer. These patients need a vascular surgical opinion to assess the extent of disease and operability. Dressings should aim to keep any exposed tendon moist to retain viability whilst not causing undue maceration. Excessive moisture within wounds, which have severely compromised arterial supply, increases the risk of wet gangrene and ensuing amputation.

After correction of the underlying arterial problem, a full assessment is again required to assess suitability for compression if any venous incompetence is present. Providing adequate blood flow has been restored, graduated compression therapy can be used to expedite healing.

In those patients who are deemed unsuitable for surgical intervention or in those in whom surgery has not been successful, management should be directed at pain relief, correction of other aetiological factors and co-factors and prevention and prompt treatment of infection.

If the arterial insufficiency is such that healing is not expected, the aim of management should be to keep the wound dry and free of infection and thus avoid wet gangrene. Simple dressings such as Betadine spray or iodine gauze are ideal for these wounds. Surgical debridement is contraindicated in these patients as this can lead to a larger area of ulceration in which there is no chance of healing.

DIABETIC FOOT ULCERATION (DFU) (Figure 9.6)

Although DFU does not usually present to dermatologists, it is important to have an understanding of this condition so that problems can be either prevented or treated at an early stage.

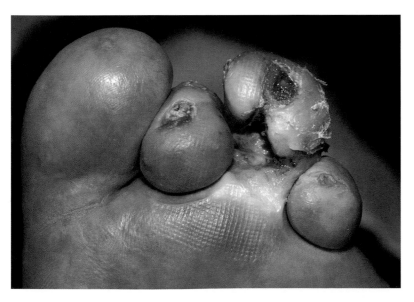

Figure 9.6
Diabetic foot ulceration.

Table 9.2: Prevention of diabetic foot ulceration in patients with diabetes and LOPS

Advice	Reason
Attend for regular chiropody/podiatry	Toenails should be kept short to avoid trauma to surrounding skin Callus should be pared Appropriate footwear can be issued Early ulceration can be detected
Wear appropriate shoes	Ill-fitting shoes will cause pressure, callus and ulceration. The diabetic foot changes shape due to diabetic motor neuropathy
Apply regular emollient to feet	Autonomic neuropathy causes dryness of the soles of the feet. This can cause cracks which act as a portal for infection
Look at soles of feet daily	Due to LOPS, patients will not be able to feel foreign bodies, blisters or ulcers
Check shoes daily for foreign objects	Checking footwear regularly prevents stones etc. from rubbing and causing problems

DFUs are essentially pressure ulcers, which occur in patients with loss of protective sensation (LOPS) (Table 9.2). They typically occur on either the plantar aspect of the foot or on the dorsum of the toes and are usually caused by trauma or repeated friction. Because of the sensory neuropathy, the patient seldom notices this trauma and may not be aware of an ulcer developing until blood is seen on the carpet. Peripheral vascular disease can play an important role in causing diabetic foot ulcers and patients presenting with ulcers at this site should be fully assessed from both the vascular and sensory point of view. Vibration is the first sense to be reduced in diabetic peripheral neuropathy.

Diabetic foot ulceration is often accompanied by infection. Early assessment by a healthcare professional with experience in management of diabetic foot ulceration is of paramount importance. Basic treatment involves exclusion of foreign body and infection, including osteomyelitis, by clinical examination and X-ray, pressure relief and treatment of any infection or vascular problems.

BASIC PRINCIPLES OF WOUND HEALING MANAGEMENT AND WOUND BED PREPARATION

At all times during the healing process the patient should be involved in decision-making to ensure maximum concordance and to enhance psychological wellbeing. Patient concerns such as pain and bulkiness of bandaging should be taken into consideration during management.

After identifying and addressing all aetiological and co-factors, the focus should be turned to wound bed preparation in order to facilitate wound healing.

Wound bed preparation addresses the local factors thought to be most important in healing, i.e. debridement, bacterial balance and moisture control.

Table 9.3: Methods of debridement

	Method	Advantages	Disadvantages
Sharp surgical debridement	Dead/devitalized tissue cut away by competent practitioner	Most effective method	Requires skilled competent practitioner and availability of equipment Analgesia often required Contraindicated in pyoderma gangrenosum
Autolytic debridement	This method uses the body's own enzymes to break down necrotic tissue. Devitalized tissue is softened and liquefied through the use of hydrating occlusive or semi-occlusive wound dressings, e.g. hydrogels, hydrocolloids, hydrofibre	Relatively inexpensive Easy to apply Painless Selective for necrotic tissue only Available in Primary and Secondary Care	Slow acting Requires regular nursing input Requires frequent monitoring for bacterial infection
Larval therapy	Using potent proteolytic enzymes the larvae liquefy and digest necrotic slough and bacteria	Fast acting Cost effective Available in Primary and Secondary Care	Unappealing to some patients Training required in application Contraindicated if wound is communicating with internal organs
Enzymatic debridement	Combination of proteolytic enzymes that break down fibrin and fibrinogen	Fast acting Selective for necrotic tissue only Best used on large wounds	Limited preparations available Expensive Preparation requires reconstitution Contraindicated in wounds with exposed structures
Mechanical debridement	Dead and devitalized tissue is removed by mechanical means such as high pressure jets	Rarely used in chronic leg ulcer management	Can be non-selective, i.e. can remove viable tissue as well as necrotic tissue Requires equipment and trained practitioners

Debridement (Table 9.3)

When the term was first coined in the 1700s, debridement referred to the surgical removal of debris from open wounds. Since then, the term has been broadened to include other methods by which the wound is cleared of devitalized tissue which may harbour bacteria and impair wound healing (Figure 9.7). It is an essential step in wound management. The selection of a debridement technique for an individual wound is variable during the lifetime of a wound and depends on the following:

• Degree of necrosis.
• Patient preference.
• Size of wound and amount of exudate production.

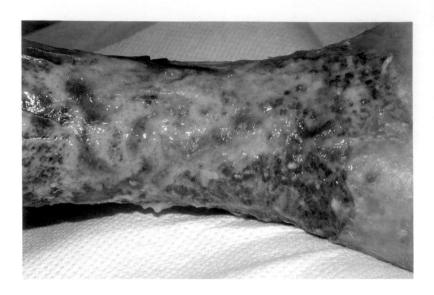

Figure 9.7
Debridement is an
essential step in wound
management.

- Aetiology of wound, e.g. avoid sharp debridement in pyoderma gangrenosum.
- Available time.
- Resources, e.g. availability of competent practitioners and equipment, requirements for theatre.
- Cost effectiveness.
- Environment, i.e. Primary or Secondary Care setting.

Bacterial balance

There is no doubt that chronic infection delays wound healing and reduces tissue tensile strength. As there is currently no gold standard test to identify wound infection, the clinician is dependent on his/her clinical skills taken together with information from wound swabs. Wound swab results provide information only about bacteria present on the wound surface. These bacteria are not necessarily responsible for delayed wound healing or infection. Microbiologists advocate that the most accurate way to assess wound bacterial burden is to perform a quantitative biopsy. This involves removing a quantity of tissue — usually with a punch biopsy — and measuring the quantity of bacteria found per gram of tissue. This procedure is, however, time-consuming and invasive. Conversely, wound swabs are quick and easy to perform and they can provide useful information in some cases. This information should, however, be used to support the clinical impression and not vice versa.

Although all chronic wounds have bacteria present within them, these bacteria are not always harmful. The state of these bacteria and their influence on the host are the most important considerations:

- *Contamination* refers to bacterial flora which has relocated to the wound from either the host or environment and which is not replicating. All wounds are contaminated.
- *Wound colonization* occurs when these bacteria are replicating but causing no host injury. It has been suggested that a certain amount of bacteria in the wound may be beneficial to healing.

- *Critical colonization.* Recently, it has been recognized that host injury and delayed wound healing can occur in the presence of very subtle clinical symptoms and signs. The concept of critical colonization has been coined to reflect these subtle findings, which suggest that bacteria are inhibiting wound healing, but not yet producing overt clinical symptoms and signs of infection.
Signs of critical colonization:
  - Increasing odour
  - Increasing pain
  - Increasing exudate
  - Beefy red granulation tissue
  - Friable granulation tissue
  - Delayed healing
- *Wound infection* is defined as the presence of multiplying bacteria within a wound, which cause host injury. In most cases, this host injury is seen as an inflammatory soft tissue response with or without systemic inflammatory symptoms and signs.

The use of antibiotics in patients with contaminated or colonized wounds has not been shown to be beneficial in promoting wound healing. Additionally, inappropriate antibiotic use contributes to antibiotic resistance.

When should I take a swab from a leg ulcer?

- When a wound appears infected. In this case, antibiotics can be started empirically and altered accordingly when the wound swab results are available.
- When critical colonization of the wound is suspected clinically.
- When a wound is failing to heal despite correction of all other factors.

Should I use topical antibacterial agents or systemic antibiotics?

Systemic antibiotics are indicated for wound infection. The choice of antibiotic should be influenced by the site, chronicity and nature of the wound as well as by previous and current wound swab results. If current wound swab results are not available at the time of prescribing, antibiotics can be prescribed empirically based on the clinical nature of the wound and previous culture results. When culture results are available, the antibiotics can be changed accordingly if there is inadequate response to those already prescribed. In general, antibiotic penetrance into wounds is not optimal. Courses of 10–14 days are usually required for wound infection.

Numerous topical antibacterial agents are now available in a plethora of wound dressings (Figure 9.8). These should be considered for use in wounds in which critical colonization is suspected, or in chronic wounds, which are failing to heal despite correction of all causes and co-factors. Antibacterial agents should be used for a maximum of 2 to 4 weeks. Preparations with neomycin and other potential sensitizers should be avoided where at all possible, particularly in venous leg ulceration. In recent years, iodine and silver have made a comeback, such that these agents are now found combined with many types of dressing. Both silver and iodine are bactericidal. By acting on three different mechanisms within the bacteria, bacterial resistance is much less likely to develop than it is with other antibacterial

Figure 9.8
A selection of currently available topical
antibacterial agents.

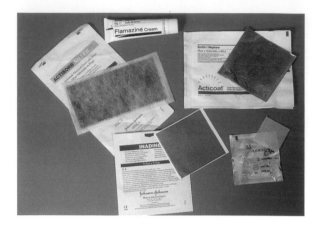

agents. Although iodine has been shown to be cytotoxic in vitro, numerous in vivo studies have shown acceleration of wound healing with its use.

Moisture control

Why does the wound have to be moist?

The theory supporting moist wound healing is based on work in the 1960s by George Winter, a zoologist, who demonstrated faster wound healing in moist wounds compared to those left exposed to the air.

Excess moisture around the wound causes maceration, irritant dermatitis and skin necrosis, all of which delay wound healing.

How do I control wound exudate?

Refractory lower limb oedema and critically colonized or infected wounds are the two main reasons for uncontrolled wound exudate. Addressing these factors will help to control the exudate. The use of more absorbent dressings and/or increased frequency of dressing changes can also be helpful.

Dressings

Wound dressings must be used in conjunction with treatment of the underlying ulcer aetiology. Failure to do this will almost inevitably result in failure to heal. Unfortunately, there is no 'one fits all' wound dressing and many different dressings are available with the aim of providing optimum wound bed preparation. The challenge to the wound care practitioner is to select the most appropriate of these treatments in a particular setting. Such treatment is highly patient-dependent, with decisions often being influenced not only by local wound factors, but also by systemic host factors. Knowledge of the action and properties of different classes of modern wound products is paramount. Wound healing is a dynamic process and the selection process must take into account the stage of wound healing. Dressings should ideally be both clinically effective and cost-effective and factors such as frequency of dressing changes, nursing time, patient comfort and patient concordance need to be considered at the same time as the ability of the dressing to maintain an optimum wound healing environment.

Classification of dressings

Most commonly used dressings are based upon five basic dressing classes (films, hydrogels, hydrocolloids, alginates and foams) (Figure 9.9). Increasingly, in a bid to create the optimum dressing, manufacturers are creating mixtures of these dressing types. Knowledge of the basic classification should provide a foundation on which to build.

Films, e.g. Tegaderm™ (least absorbent)

- Rarely used in leg ulcer management.
- Provide an occlusive dressing with no absorptive capacity.
- Useful for superficial skin tears.

Hydrogels, e.g. Intrasite gel®

- Amorphorous gel that donates fluid to wound. It hydrates slough allowing easier removal.
- Used with dry necrotic or sloughy wounds.
- Available in gel or sheet form. Sheet form useful for soothing symptoms of superficial blistering disease.
- Requires secondary dressing.

Hydrocolloids, e.g. Duoderm®

- Semi-permeable film coated with sodium carboxymethylcellulose and outer plastic film impervious to liquids and bacteria.
- Interacts with wound fluid to form a gel which hydrates the wound.
- Used with superficial leg ulcers/pressure ulcers/dry necrotic areas.

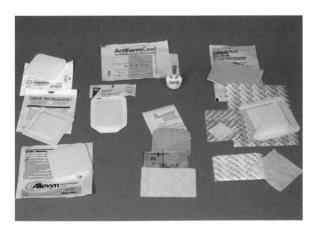

Figure 9.9 A selection of currently available dressings.

- Easy to apply and no secondary dressing required.
- Useful as an occlusive dressing when dermatitis artefacta is suspected.

Alginates, e.g. Sorbsan™

- Manufactured from variety of alginate-rich seaweeds.
- Highly absorbent. Some alginates have haemostatic properties.
- Hydrophilic gel is formed when alginate contacts wound exudate.
- Used in highly exudating wounds/ulcers.
- Wounds should be cleaned with normal saline to remove all traces of dressing fibres.
- Some require secondary dressing.

Foams, e.g. Allevyn™ (most absorbent)

- Polyurethane foam covered by semi-permeable film.
- Highly absorbent.
- Used in moderate/highly exudating wounds and cavities.
- May be adhesive/non-adhesive.
- Requires no secondary dressings.

Other dressings:

Charcoal dressings, e.g. Clinisorb®

- Charcoal fibres manufactured to become microporous cloth sheets.
- Used to control odour in malodorous wounds.
- Odour levels are reduced by activated charcoal and, in some cases, charcoal absorbs bacteria and wound toxins.
- Some dressings require primary dressing.

Non-adherent dressings for fragile skin, e.g. Mepitel®

- Soft silicone dressing with skin-friendly adhesive.
- Available as wound contact layer or with polyurethane foam backing.
- Used for non-exudating to moderately exudating wounds.
- Has the ability to conform to awkward areas.
- Useful for fragile areas of skin in blistering disorders such as pemphigus, pemphigoid and epidermolysis bullosa.

Why is the wound failing to heal?

When wounds fail to heal, the clinician must question whether the diagnosis and treatment are correct. Skin cancer developing in the edge of a wound does not always have a characteristic rolled edge. A high index of suspicion and a low threshold for biopsying wounds should be adopted if wounds fail to heal in the expected timeframe. Objective measurements of wounds should be taken at each review to allow progress to be monitored. Correct treatment should address the underlying cause of the ulcer as well as co-factors that may hinder healing. If the wound fails to heal despite correct diagnosis and treatment, patient concordance must be considered.

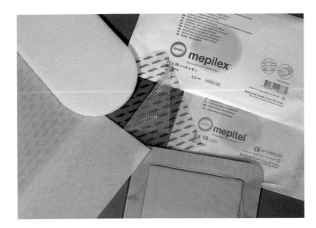

Figure 9.10
Wound dressings used for fragile skin.

BLISTERING DISEASES

Management of superficial ulceration secondary to blistering diseases follows all principles of wound healing management. Where possible, the underlying aetiology should be identified and addressed. To facilitate healing, blistered areas should be kept free of infection and pain relief should be addressed. Slitting of blisters and allowing release of fluid can help relieve discomfort and will also allow identification of new blistered areas. Where possible, blisters should not be deroofed. Necrotic skin overlying the denuded area acts as a protective layer, which is thought to impede bacterial invasion. Low adherent silicone dressings, e.g. Mepitel®/Mepilex®, are recommended for painful, raw areas (Figure 9.10). For pain relief on larger sensitive areas, hydrogel sheets can be useful. Blisters on the legs of elderly patients may heal quicker if pedal oedema is reduced. In more severe cases, the use of pressure-relieving mattresses will help to reduce friction and shear.

Further reading

Dettaan B, Ellis H, Wilkes M. The role of infection on wound healing. Surg Gynecol Obstet 1974; 138:693–700.

Dow G. Infection in chronic wounds. In: Krasner DL, Rodeheaver GT, Sibbald RG, eds. Chronic wound care: A clinical source book for healthcare professionals. 3rd edn. Wayne, PA: HMP Communications; 2001:343–356.

European Wound Management Association. Position document. Understanding compression therapy. London: Medical Education Partnership; 2003.

Mekkes JR, Loots MAM, van der Wal AC, et al. Causes, investigation and treatment of leg ulceration. Br J Dermatol 2003; 148:388–401.

Morgan DA. Formulary of wound management products. A guide for healthcare staff. 8th edn. Surrey, England: Euromed Communication; 2000.

Price P, Harding K. Measuring health-related quality of life in patients with chronic leg ulcers. Wounds 1996; 8:91–94.

Robson M. Wound infection: A failure of wound healing caused by imbalance of bacteria. Surg Clin North America 1997; 77:637–650.

Singer AJ, Clark RA. Cutaneous wound healing. N Engl J Med 1999; 341:738–746.

Thomas S. Handbook of wound dressings. London: Macmillan; 1994.

Table 9.4: Assessment of leg ulceration

Type of leg ulcer	History	Examination	Investigation	Treatment
Venous	Varicose veins +/– DVT. Pain and ankle swelling worse at end of day which is relieved with limb elevation	Ulcers typically in gaiter area of lower leg. Peripheral oedema and signs of venous hypertension present	ABPI > 0.8	High compression therapy Consider venous surgery
Arterial	Ask about intermittent claudication, rest pain, smoking, diabetes, past history of CVA/IHD	Punched out ulcers — typically on dorsum of foot or distal gangrene. Peripheral pulses absent	ABPI < 0.5 Confirm presence of venous insufficiency	Vascular surgery assessment Pain control
Mixed arteriovenous	Mixed symptoms as above	Ulcer may be circumferential	ABPI 0.5–0.8	Complete vascular assessment. Consider modified compression
Lymphoedematous	Legs chronically swollen. Usually bilateral	Non-pitting oedema with hyperkeratosis + fissuring	ABPI > 0.8 (N.B. use wide cuff)	Foot hygiene to prevent cellulitis. High compression
Vasculitic	Painful, often rapidly enlarging ulceration. May be associated with rash or other vasculitis signs	Palpable purpuric lesions develop into necrotic purplish bullae that ulcerate. Look for rash elsewhere	Biopsy	Treat underlying cause
Pyoderma gangrenosum	Painful, rapidly expanding ulcer. May be atypical site. May have underlying condition	Ragged undermined violaceous edge arising from pustule/nodule in some cases	Biopsy to exclude other causes, e.g. infection. Investigate for underlying condition	High dose steroids +/– immunosuppressants often required
Infectious	History of trauma	Nodules/pustules may precede ulceration. Look for lymphadenopathy	Swab and/or tissue biopsy for culture	As indicated by investigation
Malignancy	Long-standing ulcer. Never decreasing in size	Can be unremarkable. May have rolled edges	Low threshold for biopsy from edge of ulcer — may require multiple biopsies	Surgical removal usually indicated

Vowden KR, Goulding V, Vowden P. Hand-held Doppler assessment for peripheral arterial disease. J Wound Care 1996; 5:125–128.

Winter GD. Formation of the scab and the rate of epithelialisation of superficial wounds in the skin of the young domestic pig. Nature 1962; 183:293–294.

Photodermatology

10

Alex V. Anstey and Anthony D. Pearse

INTRODUCTION

There exists a mystique around photosensitivity disorders that prompts some dermatologists to abandon the first principles of clinical medicine and to refer patients on for a specialist opinion. This is explained, in part, by the lack of facilities for light testing in most units, even in teaching hospitals. At the other end of the spectrum is the uninformed and inexperienced clinician who is prepared to have a go at managing even the most complex and difficult photosensitivity syndromes without seeking specialist input. The ideal is found somewhere between these two extremes. Clinicians who refer on without attempting to get to grips with patients with photosensitivity should not forget that in most cases of photosensitivity, the diagnosis is made from a careful history, examination and a small number of simple (and widely available) investigations. Those clinicians who seldom or never refer on to specialist centres for investigation and monochromator light testing should not forget that in some cases, effective management of photosensitivity can only be achieved by knowing the type of condition being managed and the action spectrum of the disorder. There are now seven units in the UK with specialized facilities and expertise in light testing (in London, Amersham, Southampton, Cardiff, Manchester, Newcastle and Dundee), and four of these units have active and productive photodermatology research programmes. This places the expertise for investigation of patients with photosensitivity within reach of most UK dermatology centres. It also provides easy access for training opportunities for junior dermatologists.

NORMAL CUTANEOUS RESPONSES TO ULTRAVIOLET LIGHT

An understanding of normal skin responses to ultraviolet light is needed if abnormal responses are to be recognized. Central to an understanding of what constitutes a normal response is an appreciation of the range of these 'normal' responses as determined by racial variation in pigmentation of the skin and susceptibility to UV-induced erythema. The most commonly used shorthand for categorizing skin photo responses was devised by Professor Thomas Fitzpatrick, from Boston, and relies upon the subject's recall when questioned about their skin's response to natural sunlight in terms of whether, and to what degree, they develop erythema and tan. This system is not ideal, but is widely used, is easy to understand, and was validated (by Thomas Fitzpatrick) in 1988. However, studies have revealed that it has a low reproducibility. Skin phototyping divides everyone into one of six phototypes, ranging from Skin Type I (always burn, never tan, typically with pale white skin), to Skin Type VI (never burns, tans profusely, typically with dark brown or black skin). Thus, this measure is explicitly based on assessing two responses, erythema and tanning.

The acute cutaneous response to UVB exposure is termed the *sunburn reaction*, and represents an acute inflammatory response. Sunburn is characterized by painful erythema limited to sites of skin exposed to excess UVB. The onset of sunburn is typically delayed for 4–6 hours after sun exposure and peaks at 16–24 hours. Sunburn typically fades over 2–3 days, and in severe cases may then be followed by profuse exfoliation. The latent period between sun over-exposure and onset of erythema is thought to be explained by the time taken for damaged epidermal cells to mediate an acute inflammatory response in the dermis via cytokines and up-regulation of pro-inflammatory adhesion molecule expression.

In view of the poor reproducibility of skin phototype assessment, an alternative method for summarizing and grading different subjects' response to ultraviolet radiation was needed. The minimal erythema dose (MED) has emerged as the most widely used objective test of acute erythemal response to UVB exposure, and is based on assessment of a particular degree of erythema following a graded series of doses of ultraviolet B. The particular degree of erythema selected as the end point varies, from 'clearly defined erythema' to 'just perceptible erythema'. Inter-observer variability and site variability in MED responses within a patient can further compound the assessment of MED. When comparing MED assessment with skin phototyping, it is apparent that the two methods attempt to measure different aspects of the skin's response to ultraviolet B. The MED is a single snapshot of the erythema to a graded series of doses of UVB, while the skin phototype attempts to summarize a dynamic response and involves pigmentation as well as erythema.

BASIC PRINCIPLES OF CUTANEOUS PHOTODERMATOLOGY

Photodermatology is the study of the effects of UV and visible radiation on the skin. UV and visible radiation comprise a tiny part of the electromagnetic spectrum, and consist of energy released during the transition of a molecular electron from a higher to a lower energy orbital. The ultraviolet spectrum is subdivided, by convention, into UVC (100–280 nm), UVB (280–320 nm) and UVA (320–400 nm). Visible light ranges from 400 nm (violet) to 700 nm (red). The primary source of UV light is, of course, sunlight. Artificial sources of UV light include low pressure gas discharge lamps, medium pressure mercury lamps, and high pressure xenon arc lamps.

PHOTOTESTING

Phototesting is usually carried out to assist with establishing a diagnosis and in some instances may help with the management of the disorder. Before proceeding to light testing, the dermatologist should take a detailed history of the photosensitivity, paying particular attention to the following (Box 10.1):

- *Timing of eruption in relation to seasons.* For prolonged photosensitivity persisting for many months, a lack of seasonal variation would make a photosensitivity disorder less likely. Clearly this does not apply to short lived photosensitivity as may arise with drug-induced photosensitivity.
- *Frequency of eruption in relation to sun exposure.* Does the eruption occur following every exposure to bright sunlight? Does sunlight in the UK provoke the eruption or is it only sun exposure when abroad? Does the eruption only occur at the start of summer with the first few sun exposures?
- *Latent period between sun exposure and onset of eruption.* Is the latent period a few minutes, or a few hours or even a few days? This is important as it can be used to subdivide many of the photosensitivity disorders.
- *Duration of eruption.* Does the eruption last for a few minutes, a couple of hours or a few days? Again, this feature helps to subdivide the various photosensitivity disorders.
- *Appearance of eruption.* There is no substitute for seeing the eruption at its peak. However, this important feature is often lacking to dermatologists, as the patient may attend some time *after* the eruption has resolved. An open appointment to re-attend the clinic when the rash is present may be needed, or alternatively, a good quality digital photograph.
- *Relieving factors.* Is the eruption prevented by taking antihistamine? Is the eruption prevented by use of sunscreen? Does sunlight transmitted through glass provoke the eruption (indicating that action spectrum includes UVA and/or visible light)?
- *Exacerbating factors.* Does the eruption only occur following use of sunscreens, as is seen with photo contact dermatitis? Has the eruption only occurred since a new drug was started?
- *Change in sensitivity with repeated sun exposure (the 'hardening response').* This feature is commonly present in polymorphic light eruption, where short exposure to sunlight in the spring may be enough to provoke the eruption, whereas longer exposure to more intense sunlight later in the summer may be better tolerated.

Once a careful history and clinical examination have been completed, it should be clear if a photosensitivity disorder is possible or even likely. Before proceeding to light tests it is helpful to pause briefly to consider the possibility of a photo-aggravated disorder, rather than a primary photosensitivity condition. There are many photo-aggravated disorders,

---

Box 10.1: *History details of photosensitivity*

- Timing of eruption in relation to seasons
- Frequency of eruption in relation to sun exposure
- Latent period between sun exposure and onset of eruption
- Duration of eruption
- Appearance of eruption
- Relieving factors
- Exacerbating factors
- Change in sensitivity with repeated sun exposure ('hardening response')

and not all need to be mentioned here. However, the following conditions are common and may cause difficulty by being confused with photosensitivity disorders:

- Rosacea
- Seborrhoeic dermatitis
- Herpes labialis.

Less common photo-aggravated disorders may also cause difficulty and should also be considered. These include:

- Lupus erythematosus
- Dermatomyositis.

It is also helpful to always consider the possibility of drug-induced photosensitivity. The list of drugs that can cause photosensitivity is now long and includes representation from a diverse range of pharmacological agents. The local hospital pharmacy drug-information service can assist with cases where doubt persists. Finally, simple investigations that should be available to all UK dermatologists can be requested at this stage and include:

- Porphyrin screen
- ANA, Ro, La, +/– antibodies to double-stranded DNA if indicated
- Patch testing (important for chronic actinic dermatitis and in cases of airborne contact dermatitis which also affects exposed sites)
- Photopatch testing (important for suspected photo allergy to sunscreen components).

Indications for phototesting

The indications for referral for light testing are as follows:

- To confirm the diagnosis in suspected congenital or acquired photosensitivity.
- To define the action spectrum of the photosensitive eruption in order to assist in its management.
- To reassess the severity of photosensitivity and range of provoking wavelengths in severe cases where this information would help with management.

In practice, the following are the main conditions seen in photodermatology units for monochromator light testing:

- chronic actinic dermatitis (Figures 10.1a, b and 10.2a, b)
- solar urticaria
- hydroa vacciniforme
- actinic prurigo
- polymorphic light eruption (light tests are usually negative, and due to large numbers of cases, not all need light testing) (Figure 10.3)
- drug-induced photosensitivity
- photo contact allergy, where diagnostic clarity has yet to be achieved
- difficult photo-aggravated dermatoses, where the diagnosis remains unclear or uncertain.

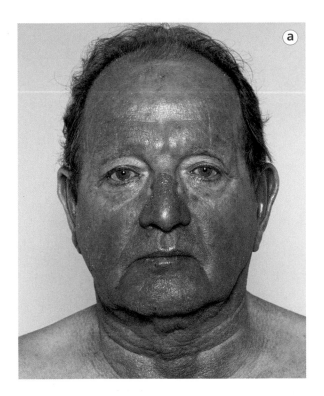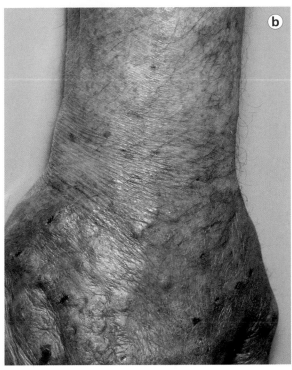

Figure 10.1
Chronic actinic dermatitis/photosensitive eczema: note the sharp cut-off between light exposed and light covered skin.

Decisions regarding which light source should be used for light testing

This is not an issue the trainee will need to decide on, as the light source for light testing depends on what is available at the local photodermatology unit, and what is the normal procedure for investigating patients. All UK photodermatology units have monochromator light testing facilities. The light source used is usually a 2500 Watt Xenon arc lamp, supplied by Oriel (USA) (Figure 10.4a, b). These lamps have an output that mimics sunlight. Skin exposure can be through a variety of UV filters in order to test at the desired waveband. Alternatively, the output of the lamp is directed through a series of mirrors and water-cooled lenses into a monochromator and then directed onto the skin (usually the back) via a liquid light guide. The monochromator is a precision optical device designed to fractionate the light to allow exposure to a clearly defined waveband. Finally, the Xenon arc lamp can be used without filters as a solar simulator, where light exposure includes UVB, UVA, visible light and infra red. Such a configuration may be desirable for photo provocation testing.

DOSIMETRY

Dosimetry from the monochromator light-testing equipment is determined at each usage by a specially calibrated thermopile. This is a piece of equipment designed to convert the

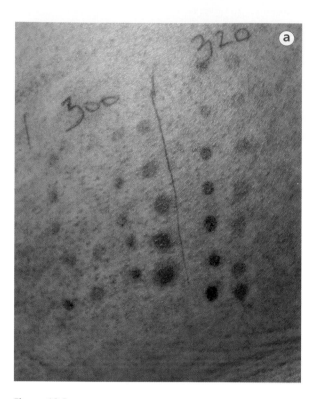
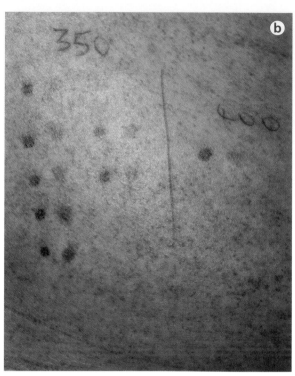

Figure 10.2
Monochromator light test reactions seen at 24 hours after irradiation in chronic actinic dermatitis, demonstrating low MEDs and therefore a sensitivity to UVR at 320, 350 and 400 nm (UVA).

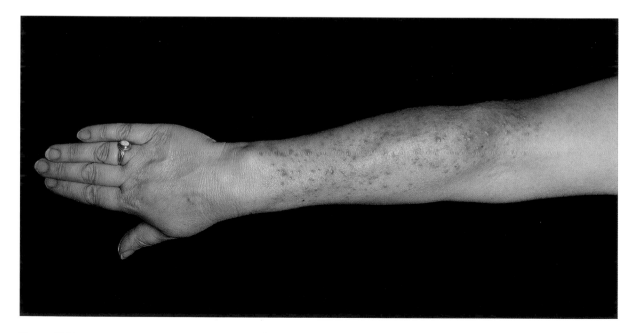

Figure 10.3
Papular, erythematous rash seen on light exposed skin of a patient with polymorphic light eruption.

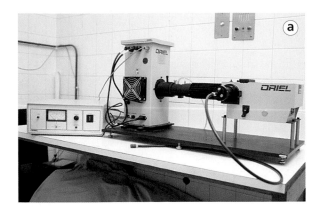 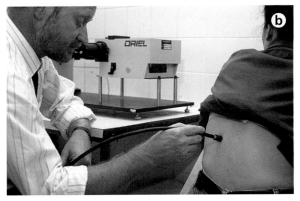

Figure 10.4
(a) A monochromator light testing system. (b) Ultraviolet radiation is delivered to the patient's skin using a flexible liquid light guide.

energy within the light into an electrical signal. Providing this device has been accurately calibrated, it is then possible to determine the output of the light-testing equipment at each wavelength (Joules/cm^2).

Wavelength

The wavelengths tested vary according to the photodermatology unit. It is commonest practice to test at a range of wavelengths within the UVB and UVA spectrum with testing in the visible range if indicated. For example, a light testing sequence may include UV exposures at 300 nm, 320 nm, 350 nm, 370 nm and 400 nm. Patients suspected of sensitivity within the visible spectrum (for example, in chronic actinic dermatitis, solar urticaria or the cutaneous porphyrias) would usually also be tested to one or both of the following wavelengths: 450 nm, 500 nm.

Dose ranges

The dose ranges used vary between the photodermatology units, and are determined by what is perceived as a 'normal' response locally. Ideally such 'normal' responses should be determined by light testing a range of patients of different skin phototype without a history of photosensitivity. In practice, this would be enormously time-consuming and, to date, has not been carried out. The range for UVB is selected to ensure that the local population of 'normals' have a MED (see earlier text) that falls in the middle of the range. In practice, 8 or 10 doses of ultraviolet light may be given at 300 nm and also at 320 nm. For UVA the dose range is selected to identify abnormal responses only. Many 'normals' require a large dose of UVA to produce an erythemal response at 24 hours, which is time-consuming and unnecessary. Thus a dose range is selected at 350 nm, 370 nm and 400 nm which is negative in normals but if positive represents an abnormal response. Testing within the visible range usually consists of a single dose at each wavelength, where a positive response (i.e. erythema at 24 hours) is abnormal, and no response is normal.

Ability to administer metered UV exposure then read and record responses

There are four situations where trainees should be able to administer metered UV exposure as a test of cutaneous responses. These are:

- Minimal erythema dose (MED) testing
- Minimal phototoxic dose (MPD) testing
- Monochromator light testing
- Photo provocation testing.

Training in MED testing and MPD testing should be available from the phototherapy nurse in the trainee's local UV-therapy unit. The reasons for testing patients' MED before starting UVB treatment are as follows:

- The starting dose for each patient is correctly determined avoiding the risk of under- or over-dosage at the start of the course of phototherapy.
- Underlying photosensitivity which had failed to be identified in the dermatology clinic (such as idiopathic photodermatosis or drug-induced phototoxicity) can be identified before treatment is commenced.

Similarly, MPD testing (minimal phototoxic dose) for PUVA also allows identification of the correct starting dose for UVA in a PUVA regimen, and may be of benefit in identifying unexpected photosensitivity. It is not necessary for trainees to become experienced in the method of monochromator light testing or photo provocation testing. However, trainees should observe these procedures in at least one patient, and should administer the UV (under supervision) in another patient.

Interpretation of photo test reactions

As with patch testing, interpretation of results of photo tests requires experience and is not always simple or straightforward. Of paramount importance is the interpretation of responses in the context of the detailed history and investigations that have already been obtained. For example, with solar urticaria the history is usually clear and the diagnosis can be made with confidence before the photo tests. Immediate weal-and-flare responses to the photo tests confirm the diagnosis, usually fading in a few hours, with normal erythemal responses at 24 hours (Figure 10.5). The tests in this situation confirm the clinical diagnosis, but also define the action spectrum. This is important as some patients with solar urticaria are sensitive to visible light as well as UV and will not be adequately protected with conventional sunscreens (which provide little protection within the visible part of the spectrum). In contrast, a minority of patients with solar urticaria fail to urticate with monochromator light testing despite a clear history and clinical features that are consistent with this diagnosis. This may be due to concomitant taking of antihistamines at the time of the light tests, but may sometimes occur without any obvious explanation. Interestingly, such patients often respond to photo provocation testing. Ideally, trainees should attend a number of photodermatology clinics in order to gain experience in the ability to read and interpret photo test reactions.

PATIENT COUNSELLING FOLLOWING LIGHT TESTING

The light tests in isolation seldom provide the diagnosis. However, light tests are usually only performed once a detailed history and examination have been completed and following the investigations described earlier in this chapter. Therefore the light testing usually concludes the investigations and in most cases is followed by a diagnosis and plan of management. Ideally, patient counselling should include a number of specific components (Box 10.2).

Detailed information concerning the clinical features and management of the congenital and acquired photodermatoses is beyond the remit of this chapter. Such information is available from a number of authoritative dermatology textbooks (see Further reading). Patient information on photodermatoses is available from all of the photodermatology

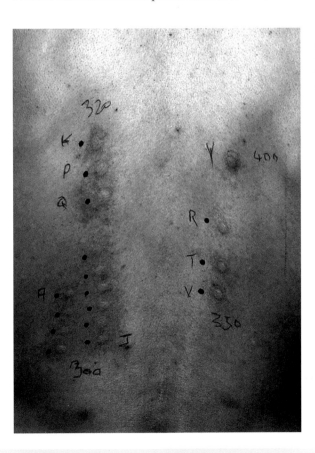

Figure 10.5
Solar urticaria: Weal and flare reactions seen within minutes of monochromator light testing a patient to UVR at 300, 320, 350 and 400 nm. These reactions typically fade within 1–2 hours.

Box 10.2: Patient counselling after light testing

- The diagnosis
- Verbal explanation about the diagnosis
- Written information about the diagnosis in the form of a patient information sheet or website
- Management plan
- Copy of letter to referring doctor summarizing above
- Review appointment (with referring doctor)

units in the UK. In addition, the British Association of Dermatologists website (www.bad.org.uk/patients) has patient information on the following photodermatoses:

- Polymorphic light eruption.
- Erythropoietic protoporphyria.
- Solar urticaria (mentioned briefly in urticaria and angio-oedema patient information leaflet).

There are other useful websites for xeroderma pigmentosum (www.xpsupportgroup.org.uk) and porphyria (www.porphyria.org.uk).

The range and diversity of the photodermatoses mean that 'counselling' requirements differ. For example, with polymorphic light eruption a simple explanation of the disorder and its management may suffice. For chronic actinic dermatitis a more detailed explanation is usually required, particularly in the elderly who may have difficulty understanding the nature of the condition and the need for sun avoidance and photo protection. It is helpful with the elderly if a relative is present to ensure that the detail of the explanation is fully understood. Similarly, in children with photodermatoses the 'counselling' is given to the parents, usually with the child in attendance. For severe congenital photosensitivity syndromes such as xeroderma pigmentosum or congenital erythropoietic porphyria, a long consultation should be anticipated, ideally in conjunction with a paediatrician and a geneticist. Such multidisciplinary representation ensures that sufficient expertise is present to provide the family with a clear understanding of the disorder, its implications, the management plan and the prognosis. It also avoids the 'experts' inadvertently contradicting each other, as may occur with a series of individual consultations.

PHOTOPATCH TESTING

Photopatch testing is a tool for evaluating cutaneous reactions caused by photo contact allergens. Fortunately, only a small number of substances cause photo contact allergy. In the 1960s, a large number of cases of cutaneous photosensitivity were seen in patients who had used soaps containing halogenated salicyanilides as antibacterial agents. In 1962 Wilkinson[1] identified the cause of the problem following an epidemic in a local factory where workers were supplied with soap containing the offending compound. The removal of halogenated salicyanilides from soap led to the resolution of this problem, but not before many patients had developed photosensitivity. Musk ambrette was another notorious photo contact allergen in the following decade. It was used as a fragrance fixative in cosmetic products and also in a higher concentration as an aftershave. It was also included in soaps, hair sprays, furniture polish, and even some sweets and foods. Once it was identified as a potent photo contact allergen, musk ambrette was withdrawn and the problem resolved. It is now prohibited by law from being used in Europe, but continues to be used in cosmetics and toiletries originating from China and the Far East.

The main area where photo contact allergy continues to cause problems is with some organic sunscreen compounds, and even this is now rare and declining. Usage of sunscreen compounds in toiletries and cosmetics led to a dramatic increase in exposure of patients to these agents. Contact and photo contact allergy to some compounds became a problem as a result, but once this was realized and the relevant organic UV filters were withdrawn, the frequency of allergic cases declined. There is now more stringent legislation in place designed to ensure that new compounds for use in the cosmetic and toiletry industries are more comprehensively evaluated to avoid future epidemics to potential photo allergens.

Indications for photopatch testing

Photopatch testing should be reserved for cases of suspected photosensitivity where the history suggests (or where it can not be ruled out) photo contact allergic dermatitis. This is a lengthy and time-consuming investigation. Furthermore, as photo contact allergic dermatitis is now uncommon, photopatch tests are usually negative. Thus, this test should be reserved where there is a high index of suspicion for this diagnosis. It may also be carried out in patients where a low index of suspicion for photo contact allergy exists, but where the history is confusing or ambiguous and the other tests have failed to clarify the diagnosis.

The commonest cause of positive reactions on photopatch testing is currently to sunscreen products. Patients who have photosensitivity on days when they have not used a sunscreen are more likely to have a primary acquired photosensitivity disorder or photo-aggravated skin complaint rather than a photo allergy to their sunscreen. Patients who have used cosmetics or toiletries that have originated from outside the European Union may still be exposed to potential photo allergens, such as musk ambrette, halogenated salicylanilide or 6-methylcoumarin (also found in fragrances, but now banned in Europe). As usage of these allergens varies from country to country, there is no single battery of allergens that is suitable for all photopatch testing. It is essential to test a patient's own products, especially ones suspicious of having caused a reaction.

History and examination of a patient suspected of suffering from photo contact dermatitis

The differential diagnosis to consider in the context of photo contact allergy includes other photosensitivity disorders, and other eczematous disorders. In the history it is important to establish what topical products the patient has used and whether there is a temporal relationship between their usage and the occurrence of the eruption. The condition most likely to cause difficulty is chronic actinic dermatitis, as the morphology of the eruption is eczematous, and there may be a history of sun exposure triggering the eruption (although this is not always present as the patient often has eczema all of the time, apparently regardless of sun exposure). Photo contact allergy is unlikely in this context if the patient has not used a sunscreen. However, the ubiquitous inclusion of sunscreens in cosmetic products means that the patient may be unaware that they are applying such products. Contact dermatitis to airborne allergens may also cause confusion. Careful examination of the skin in airborne contact allergy will usually reveal involvement of the skin of the eyelids, under the chin and behind the ears, sites typically spared by sun-mediated photosensitivity such as chronic actinic dermatitis or photo contact allergic dermatitis.

However, these subtle signs are not always present, and trainees should be alert to other diagnoses in cases of this type. Finally, both atopic eczema involving exposed sites and seborrhoeic eczema should also be considered in the differential diagnosis of exposed-site dermatitis.

Decisions about which test agents should be tested

Trainees will not need to make such decisions themselves, but need to be aware that the battery of photo allergens changes with time according to the exposure patterns of patients to potential allergens. The battery advised by the British Photodermatology Group includes five sunscreens (PABA, Octyldimethyl-PABA, Octylmethoxycinnamate, Oxybenzone and Parsol-1789).

Ability to conduct UV exposure and record photopatch test reactions

Dermatology trainees should be aware of how to carry out the UV exposure in photopatch testing and also how to record the response. As most of the contact allergens are activated by UVA rather than UVB, irradiation in photopatch testing is to UVA. Typically, patients have two identical sets of the photo contact allergens applied in parallel to the left and right sides of the back. After 2 days, these are removed. One side of the back is then covered with a suitable UV-opaque sheet, while the other side (including the site of application of the photopatch tests) is exposed to 5 J/cm^2 of UVA. In patients with significant photosensitivity to UVA, such as is seen in some cases of chronic actinic dermatitis, the dose of UVA used is reduced to 1 J/cm^2. The patient is asked to re-attend 2 days later for reading of the photopatch tests.

Interpretation of photopatch test reactions

A typical positive photopatch test is characterized by a positive response on the irradiated series, with a negative response to the same allergen on the non-irradiated side. Equal positive reactions on both sides indicates contact allergy alone. Occasionally positive responses may be seen on both sides of the back, but with a stronger response on the UV-irradiated side. This pattern suggests both contact allergy and photo contact allergy. If there is a marginally greater response on the irradiated side compared to the non-irradiated side, this indicates a phototoxic (but not photo allergic) response. If there is uncertainty due to a differing response between the two sides which could be explained either by a phototoxic response or by photo allergy, repeat testing using serial dilutions of the relevant allergen may be needed. A positive response to very low concentrations of the allergen or with a low dose of the UVA suggests photo allergy rather than phototoxicity.

Patient counselling following photopatch tests

As with patch testing, the important information to convey to the patient is what they are allergic to, how they were exposed to it and how to avoid repeat exposure in the future. This information is ideally provided in the form of a patient information sheet, complemented by an appropriate explanation. Trainees should ensure that they obtain, read and understand the information contained in patient information sheets on the relevant photo allergens. In the case of sunscreen allergy it is important to make recommendations about suitable sunscreens for future use that do not contain the offending compound. This may require assistance from your hospital drug information service. It should be noted that the content of branded sunscreens is frequently changed and that patients should not assume a product will not contain the compound they are allergic to year on year. It is best for the patient to check this every year as they obtain fresh supplies of sunscreen.

PHOTOTHERAPY/PHOTOCHEMOTHERAPY/ PHOTODYNAMIC THERAPY

Phototherapy and photochemotherapy (PUVA) are widely used in the treatment of skin disease. Their success is reflected by the ever expanding list of phototherapy units in the United Kingdom. Both forms of treatment can be dramatically effective and may transform a patient's life by clearing their skin disease. However, acute and chronic adverse reactions are not infrequent and expertise is required for the safe and effective delivery of these treatments. The recognition of potentially serious adverse effects, in particular skin malignancy, has shifted the climate of opinion worldwide towards more controlled use of phototherapy and PUVA.

Equipment available in a busy phototherapy unit may include one or more PUVA cabinets, a phototherapy canopy, a pair of hand and foot units, a phototherapy comb, a UVB phototherapy cabinet, one or more handheld radiometers, and MED and MPD testing equipment. There may also be a choice of UVB if both broadband and narrow-band machines are available. The choice for use of psoralens includes two systemic drugs (5-MOP and 8-MOP), bath psoralen, psoralen paint and psoralen gel. There is also the important treatment Re-PUVA (the use of a retinoid drug in combination with PUVA) as a PUVA-sparing option. There are now more than 20 different skin conditions in which PUVA or UVB therapy are established as effective therapies and many more in which PUVA or UVB may be effective. Finally, photodynamic therapy (PDT) has now emerged from being a topic for research to becoming an established treatment for certain forms of non-melanoma skin cancer. Dermatologists have personal opinions based on their education, training and experience. Dermatology trainees are advised to consult authoritative texts on phototherapy and to be selective in forming their own concepts about the best practice of phototherapy, PUVA and PDT.

Indications for phototherapy

Narrow-band UVB is the usual form of UVB used, having largely replaced conventional broadband UVB over the last 15 years. Narrow-band UVB includes ultraviolet radiation which is maximal in a narrow band between 311 nm and 313 nm. The rationale for the introduction of narrow-band UVB was that exclusion of wavelengths that are not therapeutically beneficial would improve efficacy and decrease the incidence of side effects. The range of conditions which respond to narrow-band UVB is similar to those that are responsive to PUVA and includes the following:

- psoriasis
- eczema
- mycosis fungoides
- chronic urticaria
- polymorphic light eruption
- pruritus
- nodular prurigo
- erythropoietic protoporphyria and
- solar urticaria.

There are other rarer conditions that may also respond to UVB including chronic actinic dermatitis and hydroa vacciniforme.

Contraindications for phototherapy

There are a number of situations where phototherapy is potentially risky or may even be harmful (Box 10.3).

Indications for photochemotherapy

Photochemotherapy is defined as the therapeutic use of psoralens in combination with UVA, and is commonly abbreviated to 'PUVA'. PUVA can be with systemic or topically applied psoralens. It is most commonly used to treat psoriasis but is also effective in a wide range of other skin disorders including eczema, vitiligo, prurigo nodularis, intractable

---

Box 10.3:

Relative contraindications to UVB therapy

- Children
- The elderly
- Patient with skin phototype I (always burn, never tan)
- Patient taking a photosensitizing drug
- Epilepsy induced by flashing lights
- Those with photo-aggravated skin disorders
- Some patients with acquired photosensitivity (although narrow-band UVB is sometimes used for this indication, it is always necessary to proceed with care)
- Patients with skin conditions known to respond poorly (or relapse early) to narrow-band UVB
- Patients with cutaneous signs of chronic photodamage

Absolute contraindications to phototherapy

- Patients with past history of skin cancer
- Patients with genetic skin cancer syndrome (xeroderma pigmentosum, Gorlin's syndrome)
- Patients unwilling or unable to comply with safety procedures (those in poor mental health or with learning difficulties)

pruritus, polymorphic light eruption and mycosis fungoides. PUVA is sometimes used to treat psoriasis that has responded poorly to prior treatment with narrow-band UVB (either incomplete response, or early relapse following withdrawal of phototherapy).

Units with facilities for bath PUVA and systemic PUVA may opt to allow their patients to choose which form of treatment they prefer (most opt for bath PUVA as patients prefer not to wear protective glasses/goggles after treatment). However, it should be noted that bath PUVA is preferable to oral PUVA in certain circumstances (Box 10.4).

Contraindications for photochemotherapy

There are a number of situations where the use of PUVA is inadvisable, or even potentially harmful (Box 10.5). The absolute contraindications are the same as for UVB phototherapy (Box 10.3).

Explain risks and benefits to patients prior to commencing therapy

Explanation of the risks and benefits of PUVA, phototherapy or PDT should be carried out by an appropriately trained and experienced member of staff. In phototherapy/PUVA units this will usually be the senior phototherapist. Dermatology trainees should sit in on a few explanation sessions of this type in order to see what information is covered by the phototherapist. The implications of treatment, including the beneficial and adverse effects, need to be explained in detail before the consent form is signed. This should be

---

Box 10.4: *Preferences for bath rather than oral PUVA*

- Patients with hepatic dysfunction
- Patients with gastrointestinal disturbance and where absorption is uncertain, e.g. after ileostomy
- Patients with cataracts
- Where compliance with eye protection may be poor.
- To permit shorter irradiation times (particularly in dark-skinned patients, for patients who suffer with claustrophobia, and with children)
- Where psoralen-drug interactions are possible, e.g. in patients taking warfarin

---

Box 10.5: *Relative contraindications to PUVA*

- Children
- The elderly
- Patient with skin phototype I (always burn, never tan)
- Patient taking a photosensitizing drug
- Intolerance of systemic psoralens (in which case, topical PUVA could be tried)
- Epilepsy induced by flashing lights
- Those with photo-aggravated skin disorders
- Some patients with acquired photosensitivity (although PUVA is sometimes used for this indication, it is always necessary to proceed with caution)
- Patients with skin conditions known to respond poorly to PUVA or relapse early

complemented by a clear and concise patient advice sheet that summarizes the points covered during the consultation with the phototherapist. Patients can not be expected to remember every aspect of therapy and the opportunity for further explanation, education and reinforcement of points can be taken as a course of treatment progresses. Children should have phototherapies explained to them in the presence of their parents (who are responsible for signing the consent form). In many units, a brief explanation of the benefits and risks of these treatments takes place in the dermatology clinic, and dermatology trainees should be confident in fulfilling this role.

Consent

The signing of the consent form should complete the ritual of pre-treatment patient explanations. As with most consent forms used in the Health Service, it is not legally binding and at best serves as a helpful reminder of the need to have a full and detailed discussion, including details about possible adverse effects, before treatment is started. As it is the dermatologist who is ultimately responsible for the patient, it is logical for the dermatologist to obtain consent, but in many units this role is delegated to the phototherapist.

Define which form of treatment should be used and its delivery (e.g. local, topical, systemic, broadband, narrow-band or PUVA)

The pattern of usage for phototherapies has altered significantly following the introduction of narrow-band UVB in the early 1990s. Prior to this date monotherapy with broadband UVB was rarely used as it was generally ineffective. In contrast, systemic PUVA was widely used as it was highly effective and well tolerated by patients. The increasing awareness of the cancer risk posed by large numbers of PUVA treatments and the greater efficacy of narrow-band UVB compared to broadband UVB led to a shift in usage of these treatments. In most units total numbers of PUVA treatments are now much lower than total numbers of UVB treatments. Furthermore, the greater acceptability to patients of bath PUVA treatment compared to systemic PUVA has led to a shift from systemic to bath delivery. This has the added advantage that the UVA treatments are much shorter, which is popular with the patients and also allows an increased throughput per day. The advantages of UVB therapy when compared with PUVA are shown in Box 10.6. The disadvantages of UVB therapy compared to PUVA are listed in Box 10.7.

Box 10.6: Advantages of UVB therapy when compared with PUVA

- No oral or topical photosensitizing drug is needed
- No eye protection is necessary *following* therapy
- The incidence of side effects is lower
- It is safe to use during pregnancy
- Irradiation times are often shorter
- It is safer than PUVA in children

Box 10.7: Disadvantages of UVB therapy compared to PUVA

- Treatment is usually given three times per week rather than two times per week or three times every 2 weeks with bath PUVA
- For some patients, duration of disease remission is shorter with UVB than with PUVA
- It is less effective than PUVA in clearing psoriasis

PUVA with psoralens applied undiluted

PUVA in combination with undiluted psoralen is used to treat limited areas of skin disease, such as occur in some cases of vitiligo. Psoralen emulsion or paint can be used by neat application to the skin disease. When treating the feet, the presence of fissuring or erosions may necessitate use of diluted psoralens to minimize stinging. Psoralen Gel (Methoxsalen 0.005%) is also available for the treatment of small areas of skin. It has a thicker consistency than either paint or emulsion, and is easier to apply to the required areas without inadvertent spread to adjacent skin. It is also usually tolerated by patients with sore and fissured skin. UVA irradiation is usually from hand and foot UVA units.

Bath PUVA

A standard treatment regimen used in PUVA units throughout the UK involves mixing 30 mL of 1.2% 8-MOP lotion in 140 litres of water (final concentration 2.6 mg/L). The patient then bathes in this solution for 10 minutes, taking care to gently swish the solution around and ensuring that all parts of the body are evenly exposed to the solution. The patient then emerges from the bath, dries the skin with a towel, and immediately enters the PUVA cabinet for exposure to UVA. The initial dose of UVA (typically $0.2–0.5 \, J/cm^2$) is determined by prior MPD testing, with increments of 20% to 40%, depending upon skin response to previous treatments. Bath PUVA is commonly given on a twice weekly regimen or three times every 2 weeks. There is no need for patients to shower or wash the skin following irradiation as cutaneous absorption and binding dynamics suggest that no free psoralen remains on the skin surface. PUVA-induced erythema with topical psoralens peaks at 3–5 days which explains why some PUVA units have changed from a twice weekly regimen to thrice 2-weekly. This avoids the chance of giving further PUVA before the erythemal response of the previous treatment has peaked.

Systemic PUVA

Some light therapy units do not have bath facilities and can not offer bath PUVA. Systemic PUVA avoids the need for bath facilities. There is a choice of two different systemic psoralens, 8-MOP and 5-MOP. 8-MOP is more photosensitizing (and therefore more effective) but has a higher incidence of side effects than 5-MOP. 8-MOP's greater photosensitizing effect may be a problem in more fair-skinned individuals and in vitiligo due to a greater risk of burning. Systemic psoralens are taken orally with a light meal 2 hours before treatment in a dose determined by body surface area at a rate of $25 \, mg/m^2$ for 8-MOP and $50 \, mg/m^2$ for 5-MOP.

Demonstrate ability to follow protocols for MED and MPD testing as well as therapy

Trainees should observe MED and MPD testing in their local light therapy unit, and should then carry out these tests under the supervision of the phototherapist. Different units use different protocols for these two tests. The easiest test to carry out is the semi-automated Durham MED skin tester. This excellent device allows the MED to be carried out rapidly, with minimum fuss or inconvenience, and results show high levels of validity and reproducibility. No such semi-automated device exists for MPD testing, as short UVA tubes equivalent to the longer tubes used in the hand and foot devices or whole body cabinets do not exist. This means that the UVA source used for MPD testing is either a UVA canopy or a single panel in a UVA cabinet. Typically, a UV-opaque template is used with windows which are closed according to a pre-determined time sequence to allow a graduated series of exposures from which the MPD can be determined. This is a time-consuming exercise, and there are a number of potential errors that can occur. Trainees are advised to follow the protocol closely and consider where errors may occur.

The routine operation of phototherapy devices requires attention to detail, if treatment is to be successful, and the chance of adverse effects minimized. Trainees should observe a number of patients being treated with each of the various modalities before they treat a patient under the supervision of the phototherapist. The phototherapists have a checklist of questions to ask before each treatment is given, and trainees need to familiarize themselves with this. There should be a file of detailed standard operating procedures (SOP) on the phototherapy unit for each piece of equipment. Trainees should ask for this SOP file and then observe for themselves how closely each SOP is adhered to.

Explain the principles of ultraviolet dosimetry and treatment regimens

Ultraviolet radiation measurements are important to ensure the consistency and repeatability of treatment doses over a period of time. It is also important to confirm the validity of treatment doses by use of calibrated meters, which are traceable back to a national reference. This ensures that $1.0 \, \text{J/cm}^2$ in Newport is the same as $1.0 \, \text{J/cm}^2$ in any other phototherapy/PUVA unit and that it agrees with internationally agreed standards. This accuracy of dose is particularly important when calculating the cumulative UV dose given to a patient, as high cumulative doses of ultraviolet radiation are associated with an increased risk of skin cancer and photo ageing. Differences in clinical outcomes are much easier to compare if we know that the dosimetry details reported from different centres are comparable.

Measuring irradiance at the skin surface

The radiant output from typical UVA lamps can be measured easily with a hand-held calibrated portable radiometer. In practice we take an average value for typical patient sizes and ensure that the patient moves about, raising the arms and legs, and turning slowly to ensure an even exposure as far as possible. The most important issue is to avoid burning skin areas that receive the highest doses of ultraviolet radiation. These areas are the sites closest to the lamps, i.e. the breasts, buttocks and, in portly patients, the abdomen.

Built-in radiometers

Modern phototherapy cabinets have built-in UV dose meters, which make operation of the cabinet easy. However, these automated systems do have drawbacks and it is important to be aware of these if mishaps are to be avoided. The most obvious drawback is that the radiometers in some phototherapy cabinets measure the irradiance of just one fluorescent tube within the machine (or two in the case of a combination UVA/UVB machine). This assumes that all tubes within the machine have a similar irradiance and that the dose of UV received by the patient (who will be standing 10–20 cm from the surface of the lamps) can be calculated from a radiometer situated immediately adjacent to a lamp. Problems may arise if individual tubes are replaced as the lamp adjacent to the radiometer may have a different irradiance to other lamps within the cabinet, producing a risk of either under- or over-dosage. Furthermore, with the very obese, relative shielding of the built-in meter may occur, with the result the cabinet will compensate and give a higher dose than was intended. For the very obese, it is safer to time the dose manually with a timer and stop the machine when the desired dose has been given (i.e. override the automated systems in the cabinet).

Testing of built-in radiometers

It is sensible to test the accuracy of built-in UV-meters regularly (monthly) by using a calibrated hand-held meter and measuring real irradiances at the surface of the body, while standing (suitably dressed and wearing UV-proof eye protection) inside the cabinet, and trainees should try this themselves. Values obtained are then compared with the values obtained by the built-in radiometer. This is not a hazardous operation in a UVA cabinet for short measurement runs. *Extra care needs to be taken* if repeating the operation with UVB lamps with complete covering of the skin with clothing. Other methods of estimating patient skin dose are available.

Radiometry in cabinets without built-in radiometers

For cabinets without built-in radiometers, UV output (irradiance) has to be measured regularly with a reliable radiometer which itself needs to be calibrated regularly. The phototherapist then has to calculate the doses to be used according to the current irradiance of the cabinet. More than a basic level of understanding is required to operate such a machine. It is recommended that radiometry measurements on such cabinets should be performed and recorded once weekly.

Other methods for estimating patient skin dose rate

The measurement of dose rate in an unoccupied cabinet overestimates the true dose which would fall on the skin of an occupant of that cabinet. This is because in the unoccupied cabinet UV radiation from each lamp illuminates the central region not just directly, but also indirectly, via reflection from the reflectors of all of the other lamps, especially those on the opposite side of the cabinet. When a patient occupies the cabinet, these reflections are blocked, and the skin dose is lower than that measured in the unoccupied cabinet, being mostly made up from direct illumination.

If dose rate measurements are made in both occupied and unoccupied situations, then the ratio of these measurements can be found. Then a measure of the unoccupied cabinet can be corrected to give an estimate of the occupied cabinet skin dose rate. Thus a once-only (or at least infrequent) measurement can be used to establish the direct-to-indirect ratio (the DIR). Such ratios are found to be in the region of 0.8–0.95 for typical cabinets. The DIR can be established by using a suitably protected person to occupy the cabinet, or by using a manikin or other inanimate shape (polystyrene blocks have been used). It is important that the position of the detector is the same for the occupied and the unoccupied measurements.

Lamp and cabinet maintenance and tube replacement

Dermatology trainees should be aware of the routine for UV equipment maintenance. This should be performed according to a pre-determined schedule established in conjunction with the local medical physics service. Ideally, all light therapy equipment should be checked once monthly. Every 6–12 months the tubes should be removed and the tubes and cabinet thoroughly cleaned. Output of the cabinet may increase after cleaning, particularly if cleaning was overdue. Trainees should ask about the routine for tube replacement in their local unit. This is usually established in conjunction with the local medical physics service.

Documentation

Trainees should ask to see the service and maintenance documentation for light therapy equipment. Accurate documentation of all aspects of routine radiometry and machine servicing are essential to provide confidence in the safety and consistency of your equipment.

PHOTODYNAMIC THERAPY

Photodynamic therapy (or PDT) is the term coined by van Tappeiner and Jesionek in 1903 to describe a photochemotherapy technique which they employed to treat skin cancer, lupus of the skin and condylomata of the genitalia, using eosin as a photosensitizer in combination with white light. In the 1940s porphyrin precursors were first used as photosensitizers. PDT has subsequently found application in many different medical disciplines, and there are several useful dermatological applications. This therapy has moved from a research setting to a mainstream therapy with the licensing of methyl-5-aminolevulinate cream for PDT of solar keratoses, basal cell carcinomas and Bowen's disease. This process is oxygen-dependent.

PDT uses a precursor chemical together with an excitation radiation, usually lying in the visible wavelengths, in the presence of oxygen. The technique requires the skin to be treated with the precursor chemical (which itself has no photosensitizing effect). Using a metabolic pathway present in all cells, the precursor drug is then rapidly metabolized to protoporphyrin IX, a potent photosensitizer. The treated skin is then irradiated with the visible light radiation. The disadvantage of using a normal synthesis pathway is that it takes time to achieve an effective build-up, so the treatment can be protracted. The results, however, make this extra time worthwhile, as the chemical precursor is preferentially taken up by pre-malignant and malignant cells. This means that the treatment has a degree of specificity which minimizes damage to normal cells. The action of the photosensitizer is the generation of toxic species (excited state oxygen radicals) during the irradiation, which leads to cell death.

Dermatological uses

The skin is an easily treated organ because of its easy accessibility. Photosensitizers can be administered topically and the radiation administered easily to the shallow depth of the dermis. Skin disorders that have been successfully treated include solar keratoses, Bowen's disease and basal cell carcinoma (BCC) especially the smaller thinner lesions. In each of these skin lesions, the abnormal cells selectively take up the porphyrin precursor, and by means of the haem synthesis pathway, produce very high levels of protoporphyrin IX (PPIX), a naturally occurring component in human cells. Protoporphyrin IX is synthesized in the mitochondria and there is evidence that mitochondrial phototoxicity is the primary cause of cell death. When the tissues are irradiated with wavelengths corresponding to the absorption peaks in protoporphyrin IX action spectrum, highly toxic reactive species of singlet oxygen are created, which quickly destroy the cells in which the ALA has been absorbed. Cells that did not take up so much of this chemical do not suffer the same concentration of excited oxygen and are spared. PDT with methylated ALA (Metvix®) is licensed for the treatment of solar keratoses, BCCs and Bowen's disease. Overall the cosmetic results are much better than with surgery or radiotherapy, and it has been suggested that targeting cells for destruction is fundamentally more sound in approach than just freezing or excising what can be seen with the naked eye. Importantly, at present, there is no evidence of cumulative toxicity or mutagenicity.

Trainees should be aware that there are two forms of cream used in PDT, only one of which is licensed. Metvix cream® is the licensed product, and 5-ALA cream is the unlicensed product which continues to be widely used for PDT for unlicensed indications. Regardless of which of these two creams is used, patients should be selected carefully for PDT after biopsy confirmation of solar keratosis, Bowen's disease or basal cell carcinoma, and warned that they must set aside several hours to complete the treatment.

Therapeutic indications

Trainees should be aware that PDT has a limited range of indications, which should be adhered to. The main indication is for the treatment of thin or non-hyperkeratotic and non-pigmented actinic keratoses on the face and scalp *when other therapies are considered less appropriate*. Metvix® PDT may also be used for the treatment of Bowen's disease and superficial and/or nodular basal cell carcinoma if they are unsuitable for other available therapies due to possible treatment-related morbidity and poor cosmetic outcome. These might include lesions at sites where local recurrence will not represent a significant clinical problem. PDT is particularly effective for the treatment of severely sun-damaged skin and large, thin pre-malignant skin lesions.

Method of administration

Trainees should observe a number of patients treated with PDT by an experienced phototherapist. Trainees should then administer the PDT treatment themselves under the supervision of the phototherapist. Treatment usually consists of two sessions 1 week apart. Before applying the ALA cream, the surface of the lesion is prepared by removal of scale and crust and by gentle roughening of the surface. Nodular BCCs are often covered by an intact epidermal keratin layer which should be gently removed. A thin layer of ALA cream is then applied (about 1 mm thick) by spatula directly onto the lesion and the surrounding 5–10 mm of normal skin. The treated area is then covered with an occlusive dressing for 3–4 hours. The dressing is then removed and the area cleaned with saline. The area is then exposed to red light with a continuous spectrum of 570–670 nm and a total light dose of 75 J/cm^2 at the lesion surface. Red light with a narrower spectrum giving the same activation of accumulated porphyrins may be used. The light intensity at the lesion surface should not exceed 200 mW/cm^2.

Only CE-marked lamps should be used, equipped with necessary filters and/or reflecting mirrors to minimize exposure to heat, blue light and UV radiation. It is important to ensure that the correct light dose is administered. The light dose is determined by factors such as size of the light field, the distance between lamp and skin surface and illumination time. These factors vary with lamp type, and the lamp should be used according to the user manual. The light dose delivered should be monitored if a suitable detector is available. Patient and operator should adhere to safety instructions provided with the light source. During illumination patient and operator should wear protective goggles which correspond to the lamp light spectrum. Healthy untreated skin surrounding the lesion does not need to be protected during illumination. Multiple lesions may be treated during the same treatment session. Lesion response should be assessed after 3 months. Lesion sites that show incomplete response may be re-treated if desired.

Contraindications for PDT

Trainees should be aware that there are a number of situations where PDT should not be used (Box 10.8).

Trainees should also note that there is no experience of treating pigmented or highly infiltrating lesions with Metvix® or 5-ALA cream. Furthermore, thick (hyperkeratotic) actinic keratoses should not be treated with Metvix® or 5-ALA cream.

Pain control for PDT

PDT is painful, and trainees should be aware of how to manage this. Men seem to cope less well with pain than women. The bald scalp is particularly sensitive. Treatment of large areas is usually more painful than treating small areas. Various strategies are used to manage the pain (Box 10.9).

Trainees should observe a number of patients receiving PDT in order to form their own views on how painful it is, and what is the optimum form of analgesia. Trainees should note that injection of local anaesthetic is seldom used as this is also painful. Furthermore,

---

Box 10.8: Contraindications for photodynamic therapy

- Patients unable to tolerate the pain associated with PDT
- Hypersensitivity to the active substance or to any excipients
- High risk BCCs, e.g. morphoeic BCCs and BCCs at high risk sites for recurrence
- Patients with cutaneous variants of porphyria
- Pregnancy

Box 10.9: Pain control for PDT

- Reassurance from the phototherapist
- Distraction by the phototherapist
- Cooling fan (as the sensation is of skin 'burning')
- Cool water spray to treatment site
- Oral analgesia, e.g. paracetamol
- Nitrous oxide (used with oxygen as analgesia during labour)

---

local anaesthetic without adrenaline has a very brief duration of action, whilst local anaesthetic with adrenaline causes localized anoxia which renders the PDT ineffective (as oxygen is needed).

Risks and likely outcomes of PDT

The best way for trainees to grasp this is to sit in on a PDT clinic. Case selection is very important. PDT should not be used indiscriminately. It is expensive, time-consuming, painful for patients and has a significant failure rate. Nevertheless it remains useful in selected cases as outlined above. The main risks of PDT relate to pain during treatment, which some patients may find intolerable. The other important risk is future recurrence of disease, particularly when treating BCCs. Trainees need to gain experience by seeing a number of patients treated by PDT before they can assess for themselves the risks and benefits of treatment. On a positive note, many patients can tolerate the pain of PDT and are pleased with the response of the disease to this novel treatment, and the excellent cosmetic result that often ensues.

Reference

1. Wilkinson DS. Photodermatitis due to tetrachlorsalicylanilide. Br J Dermatol 1961; 73:213–219.

Further reading

British Photodermatology Group. Diagnostic phototesting in the United Kingdom. Br J Dermatol 1992; 127:297–299

Diffey BL, Farr PM. The normal range in diagnostic phototesting. Br J Dermatol 1989; 120:517–524.

Taylor CR, Ortel B. Basic guidelines on the establishment of a UVB/PUVA treatment centre. In: Photodermatology. Hawk JLM, ed. London: Arnold; 1999:275–279.

Skin cancer

11

Avinash S. Belgi and Richard J. Motley

INTRODUCTION

The diagnosis and treatment of skin cancer form an increasing part of the dermatologist's workload and familiarity with the management of common skin tumours is essential.

BASAL CELL CARCINOMA (BCC)

This is the most common skin tumour (in fact it is the most common human malignancy). It is usually seen on the sun-exposed areas of the head and neck in elderly Caucasians. However, with increasing sun exposure, tumours are not uncommon in adults in their fourth decade or younger. BCC is a locally destructive tumour which almost never metastasizes, but if not treated will inexorably destroy the surrounding normal tissues.

Typical appearance

The typical BCC appears as a skin-coloured nodule often with prominent overlying telangiectasia. The tumour is soft in consistency and easily damaged by minimal trauma — such as shaving or washing the face. Once damaged the surface will often remain ulcerated giving rise to the term 'Rodent ulcer' (Figure 11.1). Secondary bacterial infection (usually *Staphylococcus aureus*) colonizes the ulcer leading to discomfort and discharge. Topical antibiotics, such as Polyfax, can be used to control this and prophylactic antibiotics should be given prior to surgery for ulcerated tumours (as flucloxacillin, 250 mg PO QDS for 5 days starting on the day of surgery).

Assessment

In assessing BCCs, it is very helpful to wet the skin with an alcohol-containing swab, and to stretch the skin whilst viewing the surface at a tangent to the light. This shows the 'pearly' changes which are characteristic of the edge of the tumour. *Any* slight changes to the skin surface surrounding the tumour should be viewed with suspicion and considered as extensions of the tumour until proven otherwise. If the lesion is crusted it is usually necessary to remove the crust before the characteristic features can be seen. It is common to detect several basal cell carcinomas in elderly patients.

Morphological variants

There are several different morphological variants of BCC and their importance is due to the likely 'subclinical' extent of the tumour and the necessary margins of excision.

The simplest BCC is the nodular variant, which consists of a single mass of tumour within the dermis (Figure 11.2). This creates a very definite 'footprint' on the skin surface and clearly visible tumour margins on clinical examination. At the other extreme, micronodular or morphoeic BCCs may produce only minor subtle changes in the surrounding skin and the true margin of the tumour may extend well beyond the visible apparent edge of the tumour. The morphological nature of the BCC is only seen on histological examination, but the clinician may suspect an infiltrative tumour if the margins of the lesion are not clearly visible.

Sun exposure risk

Sun exposure is the major risk factor for BCC and patients should be made aware of this. Some patients — particularly those presenting with multiple lesions — are at high risk of future BCCs; reducing sun exposure will decrease the risk of further tumours.

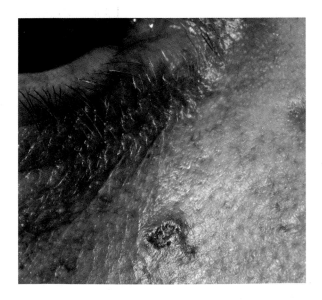

Figure 11.1
Rodent ulcer.

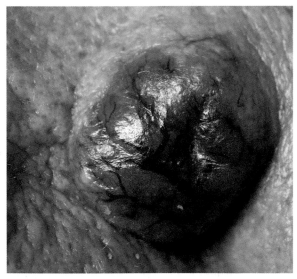

Figure 11.2
Nodular BCC.

Gorlin's syndrome

Multiple BCCs, particularly at a young age, are a feature of Gorlin's syndrome.

Nodular BCC

Nodular BCC is the most common subtype and accounts for more than 60% of cases. It presents as a pearly or translucent papule or plaque with overlying telangiectatic vessels. It may ulcerate in the centre and the patient may give a history of bleeding and crusting. Sometimes, especially in darker or easy tanning skin, the lesions show scattered brown or black pigmentation — the 'pigmented BCC' which may be confused with melanoma clinically. Some lesions have cystic centres and may mimic a cyst.

Micronodular BCC

Micronodular BCC is clinically indistinguishable from the simple nodular variety but histology reveals small nodules.

Superficial BCC

Superficial BCC is the second most common subtype accounting for 15% of all BCCs. The lesions commonly affect the torso in younger patients. They present as scaly patches or papules with a pink to red-brown colour, often with central clearing and a characteristic thin pearly border (Figure 11.3). Erosion is less common than in nodular BCC. The lesions may be confused with psoriasis or eczema but are slowly progressive and not prone to fluctuate in appearance.

Figure 11.3
Superficial BCC.

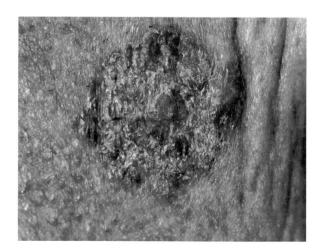

Infiltrating BCCs

Infiltrating BCCs comprise 5% of all BCCs and are characterized clinically by an ill-defined margin. Infiltrating strands and islands of tumour are seen histologically.

Morphoeic or sclerosing

BCC appears as a sclerotic (scarlike) waxy plaque or papule (Figure 11.4). The border is not well defined and tumour often extends well beyond clinical margins. Ulceration, bleeding and crusting are uncommon. It may be mistaken for scar tissue. It accounts for 3% of BCCs and occurs almost exclusively on the face.

Fibroepithelioma of Pinkus

Fibroepithelioma of Pinkus is a rare variant which presents as pink, dome shaped, smooth sessile or pedunculated papule, plaque or nodule on the torso or extremities.

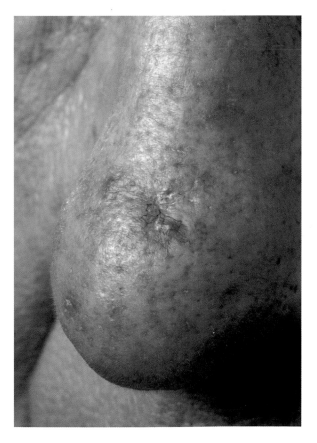

Figure 11.4
Morphoeic BCC.

Histology

The common histologic findings are nests of neoplastic basaloid cells. These nests are organized as lobules, islands, nests or chords with tumour cells aligning more densely in a palisade pattern at the periphery of these aggregates. In the dermis, intense inflammatory infiltrate is common and cleft formation, known as retraction artefact, occurs between BCC nests and stroma because of shrinkage of mucin during tissue fixation and staining. Specific histological subtypes are recognized by the architectural pattern of tumour cell aggregates and the accompanying stromal reaction.

Diagnosis

Diagnosis of BCC is essentially clinical in most cases. However, where clinical doubt exists, or when patients are referred for specialized forms of treatment, a pre-operative biopsy is recommended. When examining possible BCC, it is best to use good lighting and magnification. The affected skin should be stretched, squeezed and palpated to better estimate tumour size and depth. Oblique illumination of the tumour can highlight surface changes, such as a rolled border.

When a biopsy is considered desirable, this should consist of a small sample from the upper part of the tumour mass; usually by a 'shave' or 'scoop' biopsy. Punch biopsies not only carry the risk of displacing tumour beneath the natural base of the lesion, but also perforate the intact dermis — creating a weakness in the underlying tissue. Small elliptical incisions are preferable to deep punch biopsies.

The incomplete biopsy/excision

It is important to be quite clear about whether the intention is to take a biopsy — in which case a *small* proportion of the tumour should be sampled — or to fully excise the lesion — in which case adequate margins need to be taken around the tumour. There is nothing worse than the over-generous biopsy which all but eliminates every trace of the tumour, without giving an adequate margin of excision. This creates a problem for future surgery and a high risk of recurrence.

Treatment of BCC

Curettage and cautery (C&C) or electrodesiccation (C&E)

The soft consistency of BCC allows it to be scooped away from the skin using a curette — which is a spoon-like instrument. Curettage traditionally uses a semi-sharp curette of a ring or spoon shape. The disposable curettes which have become very popular have a scalpel-like razor sharp edge and a blunt edge — it is the blunt edge of these which should be used for curettage. After curettage, the base of the wound may be heated with cautery or diathermy to create a charred surface and curettage repeated again.

This technique is effective for simple nodular BCCs, but cannot be expected to remove infiltrative tumour strands. There is no way of assessing the adequacy of treatment (other than by prolonged follow-up) and the wound usually heals with an unsightly pale, depressed scar. For these reasons, C&C should be reserved for tumours in locations and situations where recurrence of the tumour and an unsightly scar are not of concern. BCCs on the trunk and limbs may be treated by C&C, but it is rarely an appropriate treatment for tumours on the head and neck.

Surgical excision

Excisional surgery is the appropriate treatment for the majority of BCCs, and in recent years dermatologists have become increasingly competent at surgical excision of skin cancers. Excision can be usefully combined with curettage — to better delineate the extent of the tumour, before excision with a margin of 3 mm of normal skin around the curetted defect. In the absence of curettage, a margin of 4 mm around the edge of the tumour is appropriate.

Excised tissue should be examined histologically to confirm the diagnosis and to make an assessment of the likely adequacy of excision. However, conventional histological examination of a cross-section of the excised tissue is primarily a method of confirming the nature of the tumour and any conclusions about the adequacy of surgical excision are dependent on assumptions that the morphological nature of the tumour is uniform throughout, and that the cross-section of tissue examined was representative of the entire excision.

The surgeon should avoid compromising the adequacy of excision because of concerns about repairing the surgical wound. Most wounds are closed primarily as a simple elliptical closure into a straight line, but the dermatologist with an interest in cutaneous surgery should become familiar with second intention wounds, skin grafts and skin flaps.

Mohs' micrographic surgery — for ill-defined BCCs

Micrographic surgery, pioneered by Dr Frederick Mohs, is a technique in which the entire surgical margin of excised tissue is examined histologically. It achieves the highest cure rates for BCC and is indicated for tumours with ill-defined margins, recurrent tumours and those arising at critical anatomical sites (such as the eyelid) where preservation of normal tissue is paramount. It is a precise method of histological examination and surgical repair of the wound proceeds along conventional lines.

Other treatment modalities for BCC

There are several other possible treatments for BCC. These all share the lack of any histological confirmation of the adequacy of treatment and should be used with caution in sites where recurrence of tumour is a problem.

Radiotherapy

The tumour is irradiated in several fractions over 1–2 weeks and subsequently crusts over and heals in 4–6 weeks. The true cost of radiotherapy is higher than any other treatment for BCC (but usually absorbed within the costs of the radiotherapy unit). Several visits are required and the final healing takes weeks. The initial result may be cosmetically excellent, but over time the skin becomes atrophic and telangiectatic. Radiotherapy is particularly valuable for large tumours in elderly patients.

Cryotherapy

In skilled hands, cryotherapy using liquid nitrogen delivered in a constant spray for 30 seconds after ice-ball formation and repeated after 3–5 minutes of thawing, gives cure rates for small, well-defined BCCs, compatible with other treatments. Unfortunately, even among experienced dermatologists there is still frequent incorrect use of cryotherapy with consequent poor results. Cryotherapy causes a pale, atrophic scar. It causes moderate to severe discomfort and the wound (which is essentially localized 'frostbite') is often weepy and oedematous and takes several weeks to heal.

Photodynamic therapy (pp. 190–193)

A topical photosensitizing cream (methyl amino laevulinic acid) is applied to the skin tumour for several hours, after which an appropriate light source is shone onto the tumour, activating the photosensitizer and destroying the tumour cells. Treatment is inconvenient due to the long duration of cream application, and usually painful (although there is no reason to withhold local anaesthesia). The treated skin can heal very well with excellent cosmetic results, but long term cure rates are disappointing — and lower than other treatments.

Topical chemotherapy

5-fluorouracil cream (Efudix®) may be applied regularly to BCCs and is effective for superficial lesions. Frequency of application should be tailored to the clinical response — initially applied sparingly on alternate nights for 2 months, but increased to nightly, twice daily or nightly under polythene occlusion if necessary.

Imiquimod, 5% cream, may be applied nightly, five times per week for 6 weeks, and is effective for superficial BCCs.

Both these topical treatments are best reserved for small lesions especially when multiple and on extensive areas of photodamaged skin.

Non treatment of BCCs

Not all BCCs require treatment. Aggressive treatment might be inappropriate for patients of advanced age or poor general health, especially for asymptomatic low-risk lesions that are unlikely to cause significant morbidity. Some elderly or frail patients with symptomatic or high-risk tumours might prefer less aggressive treatments designed to palliate rather than cure their tumours. Local availability of various specialized services, together with the experience and preferences of the dermatologist managing the case, are also factors which will influence the selection of therapy.

Follow-up for patients with completely excised BCC is not necessary but patient education is important prior to discharge as a significant proportion will develop new BCCs.

SQUAMOUS CELL CARCINOMA

Squamous cell carcinoma (SCC) is the second most common skin cancer. It is a malignant tumour that arises from keratinocytes of epidermis or its appendages. It is locally invasive and has a potential to metastasize to other organs.

SCC also arises on the sun-exposed skin of elderly Caucasians, but, compared to BCC, is more frequently seen on the ear, lip and dorsa of the hand. It usually presents as a crusted or warty nodule and is often tender on palpation (Figure 11.5). Unlike BCC, there is a risk of metastasis which is determined mainly by host immunity. Patients with impaired immune function, such as those taking long term immunosuppression drugs for renal transplants and those with latent leukaemias, are at high risk of metastasis from SCC. The risk of metastasis is also associated with the size of the tumour, the rate of growth and the anatomical location; tumours on the ear and lip have a worse prognosis.

Clinical features

SCC often arises from sun-damaged skin as an indurated, crusted, nodular or ulcerated lesion. The common sites for SCC are back of hands, forearms, upper part of face, lower lip and pinna. The first clinical manifestation is induration. The induration usually extends beyond the visible margins. On lip or genitalia it generally presents as a fissure or non-healing ulcer. Regional lymph nodes may be enlarged due to infection of the ulcer or metastases (harder, irregular, matted nodes). Spread by blood stream is uncommon.

Diagnosis

The diagnosis of SSC is established histologically. Irregular masses or nests of epidermal cells consisting of varying proportions of normal and anaplastic squamous cells are seen. Well-differentiated tumours are marked by the presence of horn pearls.

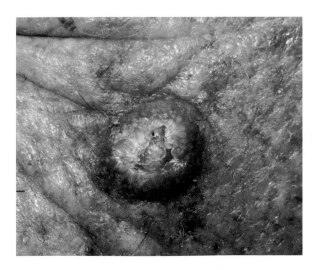

Figure 11.5
SCC.

Some facts about squamous cell carcinoma

- Most common skin cancer in dark coloured skin.
- Mucosal SCC has a greater tendency to recur and metastasize than SCC located on glabrous sun-exposed skin.
- Tumours arising in keratoses on dorsum of hands are indolent and late in metastasizing.
- Lesions on sun-exposed areas have a better prognosis than those arising from non-sun-exposed areas.
- SCC arising on the ear has the worst prognosis.
- There is a 30% risk of having a second primary SCC within 5 years after therapy for the first malignancy.
- In organ transplant patients development of SCC is directly related to time from transplantation and independent of which immunosuppressive agent is used. Lesions are multiple and distributed in sun-exposed areas.
- A distinct variant of SCC is verrucous carcinoma. It may be located on oral mucosa (oral florid papillomatoses), anogenital region (giant condyloma of Buschke and Lowenstein) or plantar surface of the foot (carcinoma cuniculatum).
- Tumours greater than 2 cm in diameter are twice as likely to recur locally and three times as likely to metastasize.
- Recurrence and metastases are less likely in tumours confined to the upper half of the dermis and less than 4 mm in depth.

Treatment

The goal of treatment is complete (preferably histologically confirmed) removal or destruction of the primary tumour and of any metastases. The treatment for an SCC depends on its type, location and risk. Surgical excision is the treatment of choice — small lesions should be removed with a 4 mm margin, larger lesions need larger margins. Curettage and cautery may be used for small, low risk lesions, and radiotherapy and cryotherapy have a place. Ill-defined and high risk lesions should be removed with microscopic control. Large SCCs should be excised and the wound left until histological confirmation of the adequacy of excision. High risk tumours are best treated by wide excision or Mohs' surgery. Radiation therapy (X-ray treatment) may be added after surgery of a high risk SCC.

After excision of high risk SCC, patients should be kept under regular review for 5 years — with particular attention to the possibility of recurrence at the original site and in the draining lymph nodes.

Prognosis

Most patients with primary cutaneous SCC have a very good prognosis. Conversely, those with metastatic disease have a poor long term prognosis. Patients with regional lymphadenopathy have a < 20% 10-year survival rate, and patients with distant metastases have < 10% 10-year survival rate.

Prevention of SCC

Prevention of sun exposure (sunscreens and protective clothing) reduces the incidence of future SCCs.

In patients with organ transplants and patients with xeroderma pigmentosum where multiple new SCC development makes surgical management difficult, systemic retinoids (acitretin) can be considered to reduce the rate of development of new lesions.

KERATOACANTHOMA

The classical keratoacanthoma (KA) is a rapidly growing epithelial tumour of hair follicle origin. It resembles squamous cell carcinoma both clinically and histologically. It grows rapidly — often reaching a size of 2 cm or more in 4–6 weeks. After a period of growth it begins to involute and heals spontaneously leaving a depressed scar.

It usually presents as a solitary lesion but multiple lesions are described as part of Ferguson–Smith or Muir–Torre syndromes.

Clinical features

Clinically, KA presents as a rapidly growing nodule with a central crater containing a keratin plug (Figure 11.6). KA arises most commonly in hair-bearing sun-exposed skin in elderly patients. The face, neck and dorsa of the upper extremities are common sites, truncal lesions are rare. KAs have also been observed in subungual and mucosal areas indicating non-follicular origin in some cases.

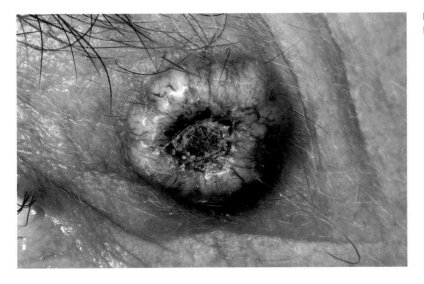

Figure 11.6
Keratoacanthoma.

Histology

KAs are composed of very well differentiated squamous epithelium with a mild degree of pleomorphism and form masses of keratin that constitute the central core of the KA. However, it can be difficult at times to differentiate KA from SCC.

Diagnosis

Rapid evolution to relatively large size, the regular crateriform shape and keratotic plug, the undamaged surrounding skin and younger age at onset as well as spontaneous resolution suggest the diagnosis (Figure 11.6). For histological diagnosis excisional or deep incisional biopsy of the lesion is preferred as the findings of a shave biopsy of KA are indistinguishable from invasive SCC.

Treatment

Despite its apparent benign nature, surgical excision is recommended — to confirm the diagnosis (because true SCC may frequently present as a rapid growing tumour of a similar appearance) and also to minimize the tissue damage which will occur if the lesion is allowed to pursue its natural course. It is not uncommon for the histology report to suggest the lesion was a SCC — the diagnosis is heavily dependent upon the correlation of clinical presentation and appearance.

Other modalities of treatment are curettage and cautery, radiotherapy and cryotherapy. Topical 5FU, imiquimod and intralesional methotrexate can aid spontaneous resolution.

ACTINIC KERATOSIS

Actinic keratosis (AK) is the most common sun-related growth. An estimated 60% of individuals older than 40 years who are predisposed develop at least one AK. Usually, affected individuals are fair-skinned, burn easily, and tan poorly, as well as have occupations or hobbies that result in excessive sun exposure. Along with cumulative UV exposure, ionizing radiation or radiant heat and exposure to products of coal distillation are also important causative agents.

Clinical features

AK lesions commonly present as erythematous scaly papules or plaques on the sun-exposed areas of the face, the ears, the forearms, and the dorsum of the hands on a background of 'weather beaten skin' (Figure 11.7).

The presence of multiple AKs is a risk factor for SCC. It has been suggested that AK lesions can progress to SCC (estimated risk < 1% per annum, latent period 10 years). The transition to malignancy is suggested by induration at the base.

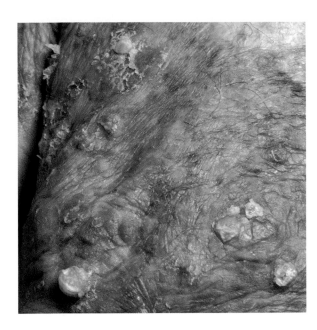

Figure 11.7
Actinic keratosis.

Histology

Epidermal changes are characterized by acanthosis and dyskeratosis with mitotic figures. Usually, marked hyperkeratosis and areas of parakeratosis with a loss of the granular layer are present. Basement membrane is intact and dyskeratotic changes rarely extend into adnexal structures.

Diagnosis

Diagnosis is essentially clinical but for suspicious, tender or indurated lesions, biopsy is indicated to rule out malignant change.

Treatment

Spontaneous resolution is reported. Common treatment modalities are cryotherapy, curettage, superficial diathermy, cautery, topical 5FU and diclofenac cream. Larger, tender and indurated lesions should be excised for histological diagnosis.

BOWEN'S DISEASE

Bowen's disease (BD) is a persistent and progressive form of in situ squamous cell carcinoma (SCC). It has the potential to progress to invasive SCC (3%), spontaneous partial regression may occur. Chronic solar damage, exposure to arsenic, congenital and acquired immunodeficiency, viral agents (HPV), therapeutic and other ionizing radiations

205

have all been implicated in the aetiology of Bowen's disease. Genital lesions of Erythroplasia of Queyrat and Bowenoid papulosis have a similar histological pattern to Bowen's disease.

Clinical features

BD appears as a gradually enlarging well demarcated scaly or hyperkeratotic macule, papule or plaque (Figure 11.8). It can appear anywhere but palms and soles are rarely affected. Lesions are generally asymptomatic in the absence of ulceration and can mimic an inflammatory dermatosis. Some facts on BD are shown in Box 11.1.

Histology

The epidermis is replaced with abnormal keratinocytes with disordered maturation and loss of polarity. Atypical mitotic figures are characteristic. Similar changes extend deeply into pilosebaceous units. A loss of granular layer with parakeratosis is typical. The basement membrane is intact.

Figure 11.8
Bowen's disease.

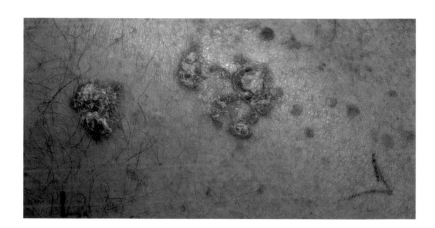

Box 11.1: Bowen's disease: some facts

- Rare before 30 years of age
- Peak incidence seventh decade in UK
- Multiple lesions in up to 20% of people
- In UK predominantly occurs in women
- Three quarters of patients have lesions on lower legs

Diagnosis

Diagnosis is primarily on the basis of typical clinical features but skin biopsy is required to diagnose invasive malignancy. Differential diagnosis includes persistent scaly macules of eczema, psoriasis, actinic keratosis and superficial spreading BCC.

Treatment

Commonly used treatment modalities are topical 5-fluorouracil, cryotherapy and curettage. Surgical excision, photodynamic therapy and topical imiquimod cream are other second line therapies. In patients with slowly progressive thin lesions, especially on the elderly lower leg where healing is poor, observation rather than intervention may be appropriate.

MERKEL CELL CARCINOMA

Merkel cell carcinoma (MCC) is a rare, aggressive, primary skin cancer exhibiting neuroendocrine differentiation. It is composed of cells which resemble the Merkel cell (MC) (this is a non-keratinizing clear cell present in the basal layer of the epidermis, free in the dermis and around hair follicles as the 'hair disc of Pinkus'). Chronic exposure to solar ultraviolet radiation (UVR), immunosuppression (endogenous or iatrogenic), erythema ab igne, and congenital ectodermal dysplasia are considered to be potential risk factors.

Clinical features

MCC presents as a solitary pink, red to violet papule, nodule or tumour on the face, extremities or buttocks. It is slightly more prevalent in elderly females and usually occurs in people > 50 years of age. Lesions rarely ulcerate and lymph node involvement is present in more than 50% of patients. It can disseminate to the central nervous system and viscera.

Histology

Nodular or diffuse patterns of aggregated, deep blue staining, small basaloid cells in the dermis are seen arranged in a trabeculated pattern. Membrane bound neurosecretory granules and perinuclear whorls of intermediate filaments are ultrastructural hallmarks of MCC.

Diagnosis

Clinically can be misdiagnosed as BCC, amelanotic melanoma, metastatic cancer or adnexal tumour. Biopsy is required to distinguish these.

Treatment

Wide local excision (3 cm margin) is usually indicated if feasible. Prophylactic lymph node dissection or irradiation is advocated by some because of the high incidence of regional metastasis. Recurrence rates are high and the 5-year survival rate for patients with regional disease is 30%.

KAPOSI'S SARCOMA

Kaposi's sarcoma (KS) is a multisystem vascular neoplasm characterized by mucocutaneous violaceous lesions and oedema. Any organ can be involved. HHV-8 has been linked convincingly with all types of KS. Immunosuppression appears to be the most significant co-factor. Average survival is 10 to 15 years. Death is usually from unrelated causes and secondary malignancies arise in > 35% of patients.

Clinical variants

Classic or European KS

Elderly males of eastern European origin are affected. This type is slowly progressive. Peak incidence is after the sixth decade and is more common in males than females. Legs are predominantly affected but abdominal viscera and lymph nodes can be involved.

African endemic KS

It is not associated with immunodeficiency and is more common in males than females. It has been described in two age groups: young adults (mean age 35) with generally benign cutaneous nodular disease and young children (mean age 3) with fulminant lymphadenopathic disease, fatal within 2 to 3 years.

HIV associated KS

HIV infected individuals have a risk of developing KS 20 000 times that of the general population and 300 times that of other immunosuppressed individuals. KS occurs predominantly in homosexual males.

Iatrogenic immunosuppression associated KS

Rare and seen in solid organ transplant recipients and individuals with chronic immunosuppressant therapy. It usually resolves on cessation of immunosuppressive therapy.

Clinical features

KS begins as ecchymotic macules which evolve into papules, plaques, nodules and tumours which are violaceous, pink, red or tan and become purplish brown. KS lesions are generally palpable and firm to hard in consistency. Lesions may start at a site of trauma and can ulcerate and become crusty. Skin lesions can be associated with lymphoedema of lower extremities due to deeper involvement of lymphatics and lymph nodes. Lesions of KS can be widespread or localized. Mucous membranes can be involved. Mucocutaneous lesions are usually asymptomatic but can be associated with significant cosmetic stigma.

Histology

The three histologic stages of KS are patch, plaque and nodular disease and correlate with clinical appearance. Vascular channels lined by atypical endothelial cells among a network of reticulin fibres and extravasated RBCs and haemosiderin deposits are seen.

Diagnosis

Clinical diagnosis is confirmed on lesional biopsy.

Treatment

The aim of the treatment is to control the symptoms of the disease as it is not 'curable'. Various modalities used for treatment are radiotherapy, cryotherapy, pulse dye laser, excision and intralesional cytotoxic therapy.

MELANOMA

Malignant melanoma is a tumour arising from an epidermal melanocyte. It is one of the most dangerous and unpredictable cancers with prognosis closely related to the size of the lesion (usually measured as Breslow thickness) at the time of tumour removal. It is assumed that most melanomas increase in size with time and that early recognition and excision of melanoma gives the greatest opportunity for cure. Diagnosis is primarily clinical and the fundamental feature is asymmetry within a pigmented lesion — which may be longstanding or newly arisen. Melanoma occurs in adults of all ages, it metastasizes easily and about one third of patients diagnosed with melanoma die from it. The incidence of melanoma has doubled every 7–10 years. The diagnosis is made on the clinical features of an irregular pigmented lesion, confirmed histologically, and the treatment is surgical excision. Some facts about melanoma are shown in Box 11.2.

Box 11.2: Melanoma: some facts

- Incidence quadrupled since 1960s
- < 10% of skin cancer cases but 80% of skin cancer deaths
- Third most common cancer amongst 15 to 39 year olds
- 80% of melanomas are caused by exposure to sunlight
- Survival depends on early diagnosis and adequate excision

Aetiological factors

Malignant melanoma occurs in genetically susceptible individuals exposed to environmental aetiological agents.

Genetic markers

Three major genes identified influence melanoma risk.

1. CDKN2A gene on chromosome 9.
2. CDK4 gene on chromosome 12.
3. Melanoma susceptibility gene on chromosome 1 (R7).

Moderate risk and very high risk factors for melanoma are shown in Boxes 11.3 and 11.4.

Types of primary melanoma

Four major types have been described.

1. Superficial spreading melanoma.
2. Nodular melanoma.
3. Lentigo maligna melanoma.
4. Acral lentiginous melanoma.

Clinical diagnosis of malignant melanoma

Melanoma may arise de novo, in an acquired melanocytic naevus or in a congenital melanocytic naevus. Very large, 'bathing trunk' naevi frequently give rise to malignant melanoma in the teenage years of life. It has not been demonstrated prospectively that

---

Box 11.3: Moderate risk factors for melanoma

- Intermittent high-intensity UV exposure (experienced by office workers during 2-week holidays in the sun)
- Regular tanning bed use before age 30 years
- Exposure to sunlight as a child and teenager
- Caucasian skin — celtic phenotype
- Latitude
- Immunosuppression

Box 11.4: Very high risk factors for melanoma

- Past history of melanoma (especially < 40 years old)
- History of eight moles greater than 6 mm diameter
- History of a changing mole
- Dysplastic naevus syndrome with family history of melanoma
- Large congenital nevus (> 15 cm)
- Xeroderma pigmentosum

small congenital moles carry an increased risk of becoming malignant, but melanomas within a congenital naevus occur more frequently than would be expected from their prevalence — thus suggesting a small increased risk of malignant change.

The key feature which suggests malignancy is asymmetry. There may be irregularity in colour — light brown, dark brown, black, blue, red and white colours may be seen, irregularity in shape, surface, edge of the lesion and overall symmetry (Figure 11.9). Bleeding is a late sign in advanced melanoma, but there may be a history of irritation, changing colour or recent growth. These changes have been abbreviated within aide memoirs such as the 5 or 7 point checklists (Box 11.5) and the ABCD rules (Box 11.6) for melanoma.

Dermatoscopy

The Dermatoscope allows a closer examination of the surface of pigmented lesions with ×10 magnification and a glass plate/oil interface or polarized light to minimize reflection from

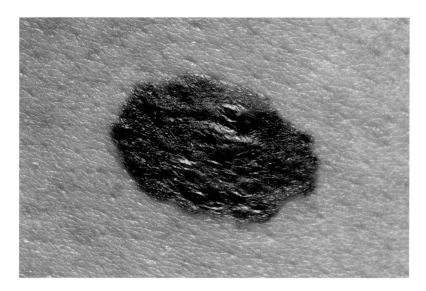

Figure 11.9
Melanoma.

Box 11.5: Glasgow 7 point checklist

Major features

- Change in size
- Irregular shape
- Irregular colour

Minor features

- Largest diameter 7 mm or more
- Inflammation
- Oozing
- Change in sensation

Lesions with any major feature or three minor ones are suspicious of melanoma the surface. A dermatoscopic score may be made, recording features such as asymmetry, number of colours, pigment structure and abruptness of border, and this score has been correlated with the likelihood of the lesion being malignant. It is advisable for dermatologists to become familiar with the use of the dermatoscope and dermatoscopy grading scales.

Certain features are found more frequently in melanoma than in benign naevi such as peripherally situated black or brown dots and globules, a blue-white veil appearance over the lesion, irregular pseudopods of pigment and asymmetric parallel linear extensions of pigment at radial margins, known as radial streaming.

Biopsy of suspected melanoma

A lesion which is suspected of being a malignant melanoma should be removed in its entirety with a 2 to 5 mm clinical margin of normal skin laterally and with a cuff of subdermal fat. It is important that the entire lesion is presented to the pathologist who will take samples across the entire tumour to determine the maximum (Breslow) thickness. When the lesion is small, the biopsy wound is usually closed primarily. If the lesion is of a significant size it may be best to leave the wound open and look after it with dressings until the histological diagnosis is confirmed or refuted. Proven melanomas need to be excised with a 1–2 cm margin, down to the next anatomical plane. If the Breslow thickness is up to 1 mm in thickness, a 1 cm margin is taken; more than 1 mm, a 2 cm margin is taken (Table 11.1).

Shave and punch biopsies are not recommended. Incisional biopsy is occasionally acceptable, for example in the differential diagnosis of lentigo maligna on the face or of acral melanoma. There is no evidence that incisional biopsy of melanoma affects outcome.

Box 11.6: American ABCD system for diagnosing melanoma

- **A**symmetry
- **B**order irregular
- **C**olour varied, especially three or more colours
- **D**iameter more than 6 mm

Table 11.1: Recommended surgical excision margins

Breslow thickness	Excision margins	Approximate 5-year survival
In situ	2–5 mm clinical margins to achieve complete histological excision	95–100%
Less than 1 mm	1 cm (narrower margins are probably safe in lesions less than 0.75 mm in depth)	95–100%
1–2 mm	1–2 cm	80–96%
2.1–4 mm	2–3 cm (2 cm preferred)	60–75%
Greater than 4 mm	2–3 cm	50%

Histology

The essential pathological feature for diagnosis of primary cutaneous melanoma is the presence of cytologically malignant melanocytes invading the dermis. Similar cells may be present in the epidermis. Other supporting features are presence of ulceration, lack of maturation of dermal melanocytic cells, presence of lymphocytic infiltrate and atypical mitoses as well as angiogenesis at the base.

Once the diagnosis of melanoma has been established, the tumour is carefully examined to determine how deeply it has grown into the skin. This degree of skin invasion is known as the 'tumour microstage'. The microstage has a tremendous bearing upon type of treatment, prognosis and survival, and is most often described in terms of Breslow thickness and Clark's level.

Breslow thickness

This is measured as distance in millimetres between overlying epidermal granular layer and the deepest invasive area of the primary tumour. Breslow thickness provides the most important histological information for prognosis in cutaneous melanoma. Tumours less than 1 mm thick (0–0.99 mm) are considered lower risk; those between 1.0–3.99 mm are intermediate risk, and 4.0 mm or more are higher risk.

Clark level

This is another procedure for assessing a melanoma. Instead of measuring the melanoma, the Clark level describes the melanoma according to the layers of the skin involved using a scale of I to V. Higher numbers indicate a deeper melanoma (Box 11.7). Since overall skin thickness varies considerably throughout the body, e.g. eyelid skin versus heel skin, the level of invasion is more qualitative than quantitative.

Most often both descriptors are used to define a melanoma (e.g. level III, 1.5 mm depth). Other important points may be noted in the pathology report (Box 11.8).

Informing patients of the diagnosis of melanoma

Breaking the news to the patient of the diagnosis of melanoma requires sensitivity and careful timing. Experience has shown that the best arrangement is for the patient to be given a clinic follow-up appointment, at the time of excision, for a date when the result will be available. It is our usual practice to give the appointment 2 weeks after the excision,

---

Box 11.7: Clark levels of melanoma

Clark level I   — The cancer involves only the epidermis
Clark level II   — The melanoma has spread somewhat to the upper dermis
Clark level III — The melanoma involves most of the upper dermis
Clark level IV — The melanoma has spread to the lower dermis
Clark level V — The melanoma has spread to the subcutis

Box 11.8: Other important points on the pathology report for melanoma

- Mitoses/mm^2
- Regression
- Ulceration
- Vascular invasion
- Microscopic satellites
- Associated naevus
- Margins

and our pathologists are told the date of the future appointment and agree to provide the report by that time. If there is a high suspicion of melanoma, the patient should be invited to bring a relative or friend to the appointment.

The prognosis can be estimated using prognostic indicator tables. It is helpful to do this before discussing the diagnosis with the patient — if the patient asks directly, it is reasonable to share the prognostic information with them.

Management of melanoma

Management includes clinical diagnosis, biopsy confirmation, definitive surgical excision, appropriate treatment of draining lymph nodes, routine follow-up of patients with melanoma confined to the primary site, management of nodal disease, management of patients with distant metastases and palliative care. Dermatologists are involved with patients with stage I and stage II melanoma. The current UK policy is to manage patients with stage III and IV melanoma in specialized melanoma units in cancer treatment centres by a multidisciplinary team (Table 11.2).

Initial assessment

Any patient with a pigmented lesion that is clinically suspicious of melanoma should have a full skin examination. The site and size of the pigmented lesion should be documented and a record should be made of other pigmented lesions. Clinical photographs may be helpful. The patient should be carefully examined for lymphadenopathy and hepatomegaly. Record keeping is very important and helpful in follow-up of patients.

Investigations

No investigations are necessary for patients with stage I and IIA disease.

Patients at intermediate or high risk of recurrent disease (stage IIB and over) should have the following staging investigations: chest X-ray; liver ultrasound or computed tomographic (CT) scan with contrast of chest, abdomen ± pelvis; liver function tests/lactate dehydrogenase; and full blood count. There is currently no place for elective lymph node dissection outside a clinical trial.

Table 11.2: The 2001 American Joint Committee on Cancer (AJCC) staging system

Stage	Primary tumour (pT)	Lymph nodes (N)	Distant metastases (M)
0	In situ tumours	No nodes	None
IA	<1.0 mm, no ulceration	No nodes	None
IB	<1.0 mm with ulceration 1.01–2.0 mm, no ulceration	No nodes	None
IIA	1.01–2.0 mm with ulceration 2.01–4.0 mm, no ulceration	No nodes	None
IIB	2.01–4.0 mm with ulceration >4.0 mm, no ulceration	No nodes	None
IIC	>4.0 mm with ulceration	No nodes	None
IIIA	Any Breslow thickness, no ulceration	Micrometastases in nodes	None
IIIB	Any Breslow thickness with ulceration Any Breslow thickness, no ulceration Any Breslow thickness ± ulceration	Micrometastases in nodes Up to three palpable nodes No nodes but in-transit metastases or satellites	None None None
IIIC	Any Breslow thickness with ulceration Any Breslow thickness ± ulceration	Up to three palpable nodes Four or more palpable nodes or matted nodes or in-transit metastases with nodes	None None
IV			M1: skin, subcutaneous or distant lymph nodes M2: lung M3: all other sites or any site with raised lactate dehydrogenase

Adjuvant therapy

There are no adjuvant therapies of proven benefit for melanoma as yet, but several clinical trials are actively recruiting patients. Most trials require entry within 8 weeks of completion of surgery and therefore this referral to the Cancer Centre should be prompt.

Follow-up and patient education

All patients should be taught self-examination because many recurrences are found by patients themselves at home rather than by clinicians in the clinic. Patients with in situ melanomas do not require follow-up. Patients with invasive melanomas should be followed up 3-monthly for 3 years. Where the melanoma thickness was less than 1 mm the patient may be discharged; others should be followed up for a further 2 years at 6-monthly intervals.

Patients with a history of melanoma should be educated regarding the information in Box 11.9.

> *Box 11.9: Patient education for melanoma*
>
> - Sun-protective measures (including sun-protective clothing and sunscreens)
> - Skin self examination for new primary melanoma
> - Possible recurrence within the melanoma scar
> - Screening of first degree relatives especially if they have a history of atypical moles

Further reading

Brodland DG, Zitelli JA. Surgical margins for excision of primary cutaneous squamous cell carcinoma. J Am Acad Dermatol 1992; 27:241–248.

Cox NH, Eedy DJ, Morton CA. Guidelines for management of Bowen's disease. Br J Dermatol 1999; 141:633–641.

Johnson TM, Tromovitch TA, Swanson NA. Combined curettage and excision: a treatment method for primary basal cell carcinoma. J Am Acad Dermatol 1991; 24:613–617.

MacKie RM. Malignant melanoma: a guide to early diagnosis. Edinburgh: Pillans and Wilson Ltd; 1994.

Marks R. Squamous cell carcinoma. Lancet 1996; 347:735–738.

Motley R, Kersey P, Lawrence C. Multiprofessional guidelines for the management of the patient with primary cutaneous squamous cell carcinoma. Br J Dermatol 2002; 146:18–25.

Roberts DLL, Anstey AV, Barlow RJ, et al. UK guidelines for the management of cutaneous melanoma. Br J Dermatol 2002; 146:7–17.

Telfer NR, Colver GB, Bowers PW. Guidelines for the management of basal cell carcinoma. Br J Dermatol 1999; 141:415–423.

Wolf DJ, Zitelli JA. Surgical margins for basal cell carcinoma. Arch Dermatol 1987; 123:340–344.

Surgical techniques

Peter J. A. Holt

INTRODUCTION

Over the last 25 years a great expansion has taken place in dermatological surgery. There has always been a surgical component in dermatology, for example the skin biopsy, excision and curettage, so why has the subject now become so important? The reason is because the case mix of referrals has changed over the years. More people are now being referred for the management of benign tumours and treatment of skin cancers. About 60% of all current referrals in our department have a potential surgical outcome.

Medical advances have resulted in more people living to retirement age and beyond. In 1971, 12% of the population in the United Kingdom was 65 years or older. By 2002 this had risen to 17% and by 2031 it is predicted that 23% of the population will be aged 65 years or older. In Wales it is estimated that the population of people aged 85 years or older will have increased by 30% in the nine years from 2002 to 2011. Skin cancer increases with age and the prevalence of skin cancer, already described as an epidemic, is set to rise.

PREPARATION FOR SKIN SURGERY

There are four categories of skin surgery – diagnostic surgery such as a biopsy, cancer surgery, cosmetic surgery and unnecessary or inappropriate surgery (Box 12.1).

As a rule confirm the diagnosis of a malignant tumour by biopsy before subjecting the patient to wide excision which may need a complex closure. Skin cancers must be excised with an adequate lateral and deep margin. Always work within the levels of your training and experience and ensure that operating facilities and equipment are adequate. If surgery is to be performed for cosmetic reasons it is essential to obtain the most favourable result. The best treatment for a benign condition is often reassurance. Poor scars resulting from surgical treatment of benign conditions may lead to complaints.

217

Discussion of the surgical procedure with the patient (Box 12.2)

Explain to the patient exactly why you want to carry out the procedure. Biopsies for diagnostic purposes are generally easily understood by the patient. If the biopsy is to be also used and kept for research then you must explain this and seek their permission for this as well. Explain what the investigation involves — whether there will be sutures and when and where these will be removed, the kind of wound dressings that will be needed and the need or otherwise for the patient to be responsible for the care of the wound at home. Warn the patient beforehand if there will be restriction of limb function post-operatively. Patients frequently think that *any* skin surgery simply involves 'whipping it off, here and now'. Beware of one-stop clinics. Many patients have no perception of what is actually involved. Surgery involving the dominant hand of a person living alone will affect their independence. Warn patients beforehand to avoid complaints afterwards. The patient who lives alone who is told for the first time post-operatively to rest with the foot elevated for 72 hours will leave hospital with a logistical problem. The patient's perception of skin surgery has been trivialized by the term 'minor surgery'. This is a misnomer. It is not a minor matter if a vital structure is irreparably damaged during surgery or if a malignant tumour is incompletely excised.

Box 12.1: Remember

If the diagnosis is not known it is impossible to know whether surgical intervention is appropriate or necessary

---

Box 12.2: Pre-operative check

Explain to the patient:

- why the procedure is necessary, and what alternatives there are
- what is to be done
  - incisional or excisional biopsy
  - curettage
  - shave excision/biopsy
- what are the consequences of not treating
- what type of wound there will be
- who will be responsible for post-operative care — the patient, a relative, practice nurse or dermatology department
- who will remove sutures and when
- if there will be reduced limb function which will restrict social, leisure activities or occupation
- when will physical recovery be complete
- what the likely cosmetic outcome will be

Ask the patient:

- to return home with a relative or friend and not to drive themselves
- to dress appropriately — for example open sandal for foot surgery, and remove make-up before arriving for surgery on face/neck

Pre-operative medical history

Ask the patient whether they have had previous surgery. This will be helpful in assessing the risk of scar hypertrophy or keloid formation. If a person is to undergo surgery in a keloid prone site such as the upper back/chest, upper arms — the 'cape' distribution — warn the patient about this risk at the time of consent. Remember that smoking reduces skin blood flow, and the risk of graft and flap failure is much higher in smokers than non-smokers. Write carefully in the notes that you have warned the patient about this and that you have recommended stopping smoking for 7 days post-operatively. If your patients heed this advice, they may actually give up smoking.

Many elderly patients are on blood pressure therapy and they must continue this treatment on the day they attend for surgery. Patients with leukaemia or myelodysplasia or patients on chemotherapy may have a risk of bleeding from thrombocytopenia or platelet dysfunction. Check their blood count pre-operatively and be prepared to liaise with your colleagues in haematology for pre-operative and post-operative support. Make a list of any drug allergies.

Many patients are now taking anticoagulants or antiplatelet therapy for prevention of vascular events in atrial fibrillation and after stroke. Procedures such as curettage, biopsy or excision with side to side closure will rarely be complicated with post-operative bleeding in patients on warfarin or 75 mg aspirin daily. The risk of post-operative bleeding increases with procedures involving large flaps or skin grafts. Knowledge of the immediate pre-operative INR (international normalized ratio) is not always a reliable predictor of post-operative bleeding. Troublesome bleeding is not usually encountered if the INR is < 2 at the time of surgery. This reduction of the INR is achieved by omitting three doses of warfarin prior to surgery. The effects of warfarin last from between 5 to 10 days but restoration of a satisfactory INR is achieved by restarting warfarin on the evening of the day of surgery.

These times are for guidance only as individual patient needs vary. For instance:

- many patients are on warfarin for atrial fibrillation, which is a 'soft' indication for anticoagulants, but patients with prosthetic valves must not have their warfarin stopped. If surgery is absolutely necessary in these patients it is important to discuss their management with the cardiologists and haematologists beforehand;
- patients on clopidogrel may have very troublesome and prolonged post-operative oozing and if possible this drug should be discontinued 1 week pre-operatively;
- patients on 150 mg aspirin or more each day will also run an increased risk of post-operative bleeding;
- stents are now often used in the treatment of coronary artery disease. It is essential to discuss with colleagues in cardiology the antiplatelet therapy necessary to preserve the function of the stent. In our hospital, patients given bare metal coronary stents are treated with aspirin 300 mg and clopidogrel 75 mg bd for 4 weeks and then aspirin 75 mg daily indefinitely. Clopidogrel should not be stopped during this 4-week period as this is a high risk period for stent thrombosis. It is probably best to avoid surgical procedures during this time while endothelialization is taking place. For patients with drug-eluting stents, the duration of antiplatelet therapy is 3 to 6 months depending on the drug which may be sirolimus or paclitaxel or a variant. These stents have anti-inflammatory and

antiproliferative properties to minimize the risks of re-stenosis, but as a side effect the time for endothelialization is prolonged, so increasing the risk of stenosis for several months. Patients with these stents need to stay on aspirin indefinitely. New stents are becoming available and each eluted drug will require a different antiplatelet regimen.

THE SKIN BIOPSY

This test is used to establish or confirm a diagnosis and it is essential to take an appropriate sample of skin (Boxes 12.3, 12.4 and 12.5). Which biopsy technique you use will depend on what you want to know. Dermatopathologists cannot report on tissue not included in the biopsy.

Box 12.3: Shave biopsy

Advantages:

- quick

Limitations:

- depth
- unsuitable for rashes, vasculitis, panniculitis or assessment of tumour invasion, e.g. Bowen's disease v SCC; keratoacanthoma v SCC; helpful to confirm the diagnosis and type of basal cell carcinoma

Remember — if further surgery is contemplated, leave sufficient remnant of the tumour to identify the site

Before you perform a shave biopsy be sure you know its limitations

---

Box 12.4: Punch biopsy

Advantages:

- quick; easy to process in the pathology lab
- suitable for biopsies of rashes and tumours
- defects < 6 mm easy to suture

Limitations:

- depth — e.g. unsuitable in panniculitis, morphoea and some cases of vasculitis
- limitations in assessing depth of tumour invasion

Box 12.5: Incisional biopsy

- Gives you the big picture. Large surface area and depth
- Useful to examine the edge of an ulcer or a rash to compare with 'normal' adjacent skin
- The full thickness allows examination of the fat, deep blood vessels, useful in suspected infiltrative diseases and granulomatous disorders, morphoea, scleroderma and mucinoses
- Incision/excision biopsy is essential for:
  - suspected melanoma
  - distinction between keratoacanthoma and SCC
  - assessment of tumour invasion

- A biopsy of a rash is often most helpful in early stages of its development when the changes may be more specific. For example, the pre-bullous weal is much more helpful than a biopsy of an intact blister in cases of pemphigoid and dermatitis herpetiformis.
- The histology of ulcerating lesions is best obtained by taking a biopsy through the edge of the lesion from the normal skin to the centre.

If the biopsy is unhelpful, be prepared to repeat the investigation.

Useful information and techniques

- The pathologist is helped by a good differential diagnosis and it is important that the histology form is completed with a sensible and legible differential diagnosis. Unhelpful information like 'rash ? cause' will probably be reported as 'non-specific inflammation'. Be prepared to discuss the patient's details with the dermatopathologist. Seek the advice of a more experienced colleague if you are unsure of what to biopsy; an inappropriate biopsy is a waste of your time and an inconvenience to the patient.
- Skin diseases may have an epidermal, dermal or a subcutaneous component. The most appropriate biopsy technique is the ellipse or punch biopsy which will include fat. Remember to include the advancing edge of an extending rash and ensure that the biopsy has a sufficient depth. A punch biopsy may not include sufficient depth of skin in some cases of morphoea, panniculitis or vasculitis. Dermatopathologists are often helped by patterns of inflammation, so allow them to cut multiple levels to see the 'big picture' by taking a biopsy with sufficient surface area and depth.
- Biopsies of tumours (Figure 12.1) are important investigations to establish or confirm diagnoses.

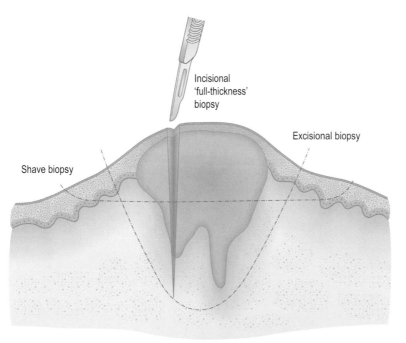

Figure 12.1
Types of skin biopsy.

Incisional 'full-thickness' biopsy

Excisional biopsy

Shave biopsy

- Shave biopsy of any exophytic tumour will contain tumour at the deep surgical margin and will give no information as to the depth of invasion. The shave will confirm the cytological type of the tumour but will not distinguish, for example, a squamous cell carcinoma from Bowen's disease as there will be insufficient dermis to assess invasion. Shave biopsies are a very effective treatment for removing suspected junctional, compound or cellular (intradermal) naevi. The shave biopsy has become a very popular technique — it is quick and easy to perform but it is important to know its limitations.
- Suspected melanomas must always be removed as an excisional biopsy to allow adequate staging of the tumour. Rapidly growing tumours such as squamous cell carcinomas or keratoacanthomas can only be reliably distinguished by biopsies 'through and through' allowing the pathologist to examine low power the overall architecture of the 'shoulders' of the lesion and the depth of invasion.

Local anaesthetics

Lidocaine

Lidocaine is the most widely used drug for local anaesthesia of the skin. Concentrations of 1% and 2% are widely available with adrenaline (1:80 000 and 1:200 000) or without adrenaline — plain lidocaine. The maximum safe dose of subcutaneous lidocaine is 3 mg/kg without adrenaline and 7 mg/kg with adrenaline. Lidocaine 1% contains 10 mg of lidocaine/mL. A 70 kg man should therefore have no more than 10 mL of 2% lidocaine or 50 mL of 1% lidocaine with 1:200 000 adrenaline. Adrenaline prolongs the duration of anaesthesia and causes vasoconstriction, two very useful properties. 1:1000 adrenaline contains 1 mg/mL; 1:100 000 contains 1 mg adrenaline/100 mL. It is seldom necessary to infiltrate more than 50 mL of 1% lidocaine with 1:200 000 adrenaline (250 µg), so the safety margin for adrenaline is high. Large volumes of anaesthetic used in tumescent anaesthesia require a greater dilution of lidocaine and adrenaline. Adrenaline has alpha-1 (vasoconstriction), beta-1 (inotropic, chronotropic) and beta-2 (vasodilatation) properties. Its use in patients taking non-cardioselective betablockers may give rise to unopposed alpha-1 vasoconstriction leading to hypertension and reflex bradycardia.

Disposable cartridges

Many departments use disposable cartridges containing 2% lidocaine with 1:80 000 adrenaline. This system has been used for many years by dental surgeons; it is a quick and convenient method that is suitable for nerve blocks commonly used intra-orally by dentists. Plain lidocaine cartridges are currently unavailable and 4% prilocaine may be used instead. The maximum recommended dose should not exceed 6 mg/kg, or 8 mg/kg with adrenaline.

Nerve blocks

Nerve blocks used commonly in dermatology are supraorbital/supratrochlear nerve blocks and infraorbital and mental nerve blocks. Adrenalized lidocaine should be avoided when giving digital ring blocks. Plain lidocaine or prilocaine should be used instead. A volume of 4 mL on either side of the digit should not be exceeded to prevent ischaemia from compression. It is safe to use lidocaine with adrenaline for subcutaneous infiltration on the nose, ear and penis.

Disposable syringes

Disposable syringe systems are now available with aspiration devices which are useful to check for intravascular injection.

Accidental injection and toxicity

When accidental intravascular injection occurs — as seen often as a white outline of the vascular network around the injection site, stop injecting immediately. Signs of minor toxicity of lidocaine includes circumoral paraesthesiae, tinnitus and dizziness and sometimes a metallic taste.

Injection technique

Injection of local anaesthetic is uncomfortable (Box 12.6). A fine gauged needle — 27 G or preferably 30 G should be used. The skin to be injected should be pinched to decrease pain perception and the patient warned about the injection beforehand. Try and introduce the needle down a follicle with the bevel of the needle pointed downwards and injcct subcutaneously and not intradermally. The injection should be slow and the syringe aspirated frequently to check for intravascular injection.

Multi-dose bottles

Multi-dose bottles of local anaesthetic are widely used. They contain lidocaine, adrenaline, sodium metabisulphite (anti-oxidant) and also parabens (preservative). Lidocaine 2% is considered more painful than 0.5% preservative-free plain lidocaine. Adrenaline and sodium metabisulphite both significantly increase the discomfort associated with the injection.[1] Warming the anaesthetic to 37°C may cause less discomfort than anaesthetic at 20°C. Local anaesthetic remaining in a multi-dose vial must not be used to treat another patient because of the risk of cross infection. Partly used bottles must be thrown away at the end of the theatre session.

Box 12.6: Reducing the pain of local anaesthesia

- sedation:
  - children – trimeprazine 3 mg/kg 2 h pre-op
  - adults — diazepam 5 mg po 2 h pre-op
- EMLA: 2 h pre-op
- Ametop: 30 min pre-op
- 0.5% plain lidocaine preservative free injection using a 30G needle
- then 1% lidocaine with 1:200 000 adrenaline, followed by
- 0.5% bupivacaine for prolonged (post-operative) anaesthesia
- check effectiveness of anaesthetic before starting the procedure

Bupivacaine

Bupivacaine is an anaesthetic with slow onset and long duration (5 to 8 hours). It can provide post-operative pain relief as well and is available as 0.25% and 0.5% concentrations. The maximum safe dosage for bupivacaine is 2 mg/kg.

Effects of local anaesthesia

The type C pain fibres are anaesthetized more quickly than the larger pressure and proprioceptive fibres. Warn patients beforehand that they will feel pressure and joint movement and that this does not indicate failure of the local anaesthetic. Motor fibres are affected later on after the injection. It is important to warn the patients who have had infiltrative anaesthesia on the face that they may not be able to raise the eyebrows or tightly close the eyes after injections in the temple region or have drooping of the mouth for some hours after an injection in the cheek.

ANATOMY

It is essential to have a sound knowledge of basic anatomy especially of the face when operating on the skin (Figure 12.2).

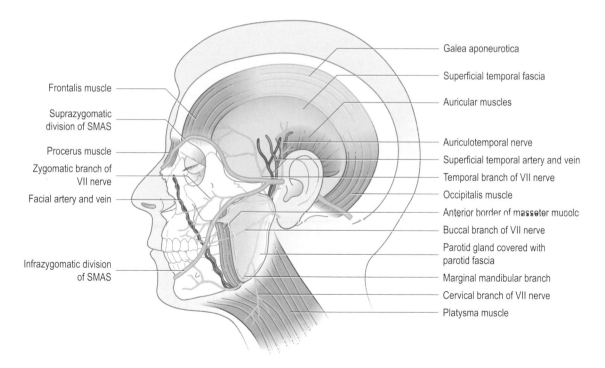

Figure 12.2
Diagram of the face to show the location of the branches of the facial nerve in relation to the fascia and the parotid gland, and the overlying facial and superficial temporal arteries.

Superficial musculoaponeurotic system (SMAS)

On the face the skin with the underlying fat lies on the superficial fascia which is known as the superficial musculoaponeurotic system (SMAS). Above the zygoma this layer is known as the superficial temporal fascia, splitting to ensheave the frontalis, procerus, occipitalis and auricular muscles and then extending up on the scalp as the fibrous galea. Below this fascia is the deep temporalis fascia covering the temporalis muscle. Below the zygoma, the SMAS is made up of parotid fascia which is a fibrotic degeneration of the platysma muscle and the parotid fascia is in continuity with the platysma, risorius and depressor anguli oris muscles. The central facial and nasal muscles are devoid of a distinct aponeurotic component.

Blood vessels and nerves

Knowledge of the SMAS helps predict the location and depth of important blood vessels and nerves.

- Blood vessels
  - Axial blood vessels and sensory nerves to the upper face arise deeply and ascend to lie in the SMAS/fat interface.
  - The superficial temporal artery is frequently seen on the temple and forehead and it lies on the superficial temporal fascia and is above the plane of the temporal branch of the facial nerve which runs beneath this fascia upon the deep temporalis fascia.
  - On the forehead, branches of the supratrochlear and supraorbital nerves run on the fascia above the frontalis muscle, along with branches of the supraorbital and supratrochlear arteries.
- Nerves
  - The facial nerve exits the skull through the stylomastoid foramen and enters the parotid gland at the mid point of a line connecting the superior border of the tragus of the ear to the angle of the jaw.
  - The temporal branch of the facial nerve exits the parotid gland and rami are distributed over the middle third of the zygomatic arch.
  - The medial part of the zygomatic arch is a safe area as the nerve has now entered the orbicularis muscle. It is most vulnerable over a 25 mm section over the mid part of the zygomatic arch. Here the nerve is covered only by fascia, fat and skin. This area can be mapped out by:
    1. a line drawn from the tragus to the upper forehead crease and
    2. a second line drawn from the ear lobe to the eyebrow (Figure 12.3a).
  - The path of the ramus to the frontalis muscle is along a line drawn 0.5 cm below the tragus to 1.5 cm above the lateral eyebrow (Figure 12.3b). This ramus lies between the SMAS (superficial temporal fascia) and the deep temporalis fascia before it enters the frontalis muscle at its lateral border.

The superficial temporal artery and vein along with the auriculotemporal nerve emerge from the parotid gland and lie on the superficial temporal fascia. If working within no more than 1 cm anterior to a vertical line drawn from the scalp to the insertion of the anterior helix of the ear, the posterior ramus of the temporal branch is safe.

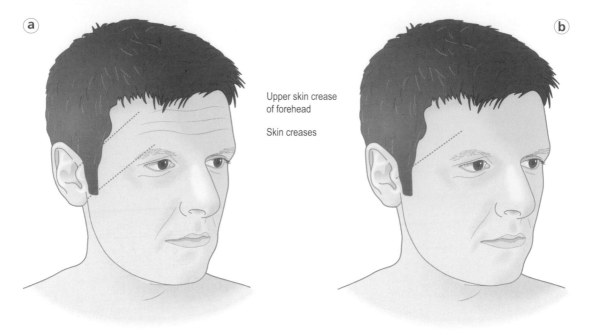

Upper skin crease
of forehead

Skin creases

Figure 12.3
(a) The surface marking the temporal branch of the VII cranial nerve and (b) the path of the ramus to the frontalis muscle.

- The zygomatic and buccal branches of the facial nerve pass medially from the parotid gland on the masseteric fascia. The SMAS is very poorly developed here, and the nerves are covered by skin and fat which, however, is quite deep at this site.
- The branches of the zygomatic and buccal nerves anastomose:
  1. just anterior to the masseter and
  2. at the point under the modiolus (the dimple).

These two points correspond to the posterior and anterior border of the buccal fat pad respectively which is seen when removing deeply invasive tumours over the mid cheek area. Rich anastomoses between these two branches account for frequent recovery if some of the branches are damaged.

Parotid duct

Another structure below the fat in this area is the parotid duct. This leaves the parotid gland and continues anteriorly before winding round the anterior border of the masseter muscle before piercing the buccinator muscle to enter the oral cavity by the second upper molar tooth.

The parotid duct can be felt under your finger when you clench your teeth and palpate the anterior border of the masseter muscle. The duct can be mapped to a point where a line from the tragus to the upper lip crosses the anterior border of the masseter — the tragolabial line.

The area where the masseter muscle attaches to the mandible

At the point where the anterior border of the masseter muscle attaches to the mandible, the facial artery can be felt. Behind the artery lies the facial vein and in front of the artery lies the marginal mandibular nerve. The nerve at this point is vulnerable to injury. It is covered only by a variable amount of platysma muscle, fat and skin. There is only an anastomosis with the buccal nerve in 10% of people. Injury to this nerve is very serious as it innovates the lower lip muscles which are essential to achieve oral continence.

Neck

Posterior triangle

In the neck the most important area for dermatological surgeons is the posterior triangle, bounded by the clavicle inferiorly, the posterior border of the sternomastoid anteriorly and the anterior border of the trapezius posteriorly. The floor of the triangle consists of the splenius capitis muscle superiorly, the levator scapulae and the posterior and midscalene muscles inferiorly, which are covered by the prevertebral layer of the deep cervical fascia which is itself covered by the superficial layer of the deep cervical fascia. Between these layers of fascia many important structures are located on the floor of this triangle:

- The lesser occipital nerve, great auricular nerve, transverse cervical nerve and the spinal accessory nerve which is the motor nerve to the trapezius and sternomastoid muscles.
- Erb's point is located where a line perpendicular from the mid point of a line drawn from the angle of the jaw to the mastoid crosses the posterior border of the sternomastoid muscle. These aforementioned nerves lie within an area 1 cm above and below this point.
- The spinal accessory nerve runs on the floor of the posterior triangle from approximately the junction of the upper one third/lower two thirds of the sternomastoid muscle descending approximately obliquely to leave the triangle at the junction of the middle/lower third of the trapezius muscle.

The structures in the posterior triangle are covered by skin, fat and the superficial layer of the deep cervical fascia which ensheaves the trapezius muscle posteriorly and the sternomastoid muscle anteriorly.

These structures are safe providing the fascia is not breached. This can occur when attempting to remove an epidermoid cyst in the posterior triangle or excising a deeply invasive malignant tumour. Damage to the spinal accessory nerve will result in shoulder drop due to paralysis of the trapezius muscle.

Ulnar and common peroneal nerves

Other motor nerves rarely encountered by dermatological surgeons are the ulnar nerve at the elbow where it runs 1 cm below and lateral to the medial epicondyle of the humerus and the common peroneal nerve (lateral popliteal nerve) as it winds around the head of the fibula. The nerves at these points are very superficial.

HAEMOSTASIS

Haemostasis for surface wounds

Styptics

For haemostasis of superficial wounds, such as shave excision or curettage, a styptic such as 20% aluminium chloride in 70% isopropyl alcohol can be used. This acts as a protein precipitating agent. Driclor is an alternative. Older agents such as silver nitrate and Monsel's solution (ferric subsulphate) are seldom used now because of the small risk of pigment tattooing.

Electrocautery

Electrocautery is a useful haemostat — a current passing through a high resistance metal such as platinum produces heat — the cautery tip is like a toaster or soldering iron.

Calibration of instruments do not conform to a standardized power output. The best working temperature is 'below the red glow' which corresponds to 60–80°C. The tip should be applied very lightly to the wound surface which should be pressed dry with gauze immediately before contact.

It is important that the contact time must be very brief to reduce injury from transmitted heat. Higher temperatures (100°C) cause water in the tissues to steam; at 350°C, the tissue carbonizes and at 500°C the tissue will catch fire. It is important not to use alcohol-based antiseptics in the vicinity of cautery instruments (or sparking from diathermy instruments). It is not difficult to set fire to your patient.

Cautery tips must be sterilized between patients, and handles and leads covered with disposable sleeves to prevent contamination with blood.

Diathermy

Diathermy is another technique for haemostasis.

- Surgical diathermy generates heat by:
  - resistance to current which passes through the tissues;
  - duration of application of the current (proportional to the square of the current);
  - current density — which is inversely proportional to the surface area of the electrosurgery tip; and
  - heat from sparking — the temperature of an electric spark can be as high as 1000°C.
- Sparking is achieved by activating the diathermy tip without making contact with the skin surface. This is known as *electrofulguration* (L fulgur = lightening). This technique may result in slight surface damage and can cause slight scarring. The deeper tissues are not damaged because charring acts as an insulating barrier.
- Direct contact with the skin and the diathermy tip results in *electrodesiccation*. The heat generated from the current and the current density produces heating (and therefore injury) at a deeper level than is achieved with fulguration.

With instruments such as the Hyfrecator, fulguration or desiccation is achieved without a dispersive electrode. The patient acts as a capacitor with the ground, shedding free electrons from the skin surface to the air, the couch, the operator and the assistant before going to ground. It is sometimes possible for the operator or the nurse to discern a shock or tingle if the patient is touched lightly. This is more likely at higher power settings or if the hand is ungloved or the tip of the finger is in contact (small surface area such as a fingertip allows discharge at a point like a lightning conductor) with the patient. The operator and the assistant should make contact with the flat of the hand rather than the fingertip. Doubling the surface area will half the current density and reduce the heat by a quarter.

Haemostasis for deeper wounds

Bleeding from the depth of a wound following excision is best dealt with immediately by firm pressure around the edge of the wound. This allows the bleeding to stop and the vessel to be identified. The vessel can then be sealed with diathermy and if this is not successful the vessel can be tied with an absorbable suture using a figure of eight knot.

Electrocoagulation

With classical electrocoagulation an indifferent (neutral) electrode is attached to the patient. This forms a ready current run-off, and so the potential difference between the machine and the patient in the circuit is greater than if no plate is used. Lower voltages are therefore required while the current flow is increased. The current of injury applied to the tissue by the forceps may 'channel down' the vessel and cause greater tissue necrosis.

Instruments now used widely for electrocoagulation in skin surgery do not have a dispersive electrode and are the 'bipolar' type. The sides of the coagulation forceps are insulated and AC current flows between the tips of the forceps which are grasping the tissue. The current density is high and the distance between the tip is small so the tissue resistance is lowered. Tissue damage is much more localized.

Complications of electrosurgery instruments

- Burns due to :
  - poor surface contact with the dispersive electrode;
  - inadvertent contact with the earth or ground through metal on the operating table; and
  - fire risk from alcohol-based antiseptics.
- Pacemaker interference
  - The sensing function of a demand pacemaker may pick up stray electromagnetic radiation (EMR) from electrosurgical apparatus and interpret this as cardiac muscle myopotential — this in turn could inhibit generator function.
  - In practice very few problems are encountered because modern pacemakers are insulated with titanium which filters and screens stray EMR from machines such as microwaves and shavers.

If a person has a pacemaker:

> Use short bursts of activity (less than 5 seconds).
> Avoid using the active electrode over the precordium in a patient with a pacemaker or on the skin over the pacemaker power source.
> Turn the pacemaker to fixed rate.
> If in any doubt speak to the technical support team in the Cardiology Department.

NEEDLES AND SUTURES

There are a great many to choose from and you are advised to read one of the standard texts or workshop manuals for further information.[2]

Needles

- The shape of the needles is commonly $\frac{3}{8}$ circle.
- Compound curve (J-shape) needles are particularly useful in placing subcuticular buried stitches in confined areas.
- Small needles are 12 mm in length and are often attached to fine sutures used on the face.
- Needles of 19 mm are used for the trunk and limbs.
- Some sutures are attached to large 25 or 29 mm needles and are useful if large bites of skin are needed.
- Modern needles are usually manufactured with either the inner or the outer surface of the curve honed to a sharp edge. These are known respectively as cutting or reverse cutting needles. Reverse cutting needles are best for skin surgery as this prevents the needle track from cutting in towards the wound edge during the passage of the needle.
- 'P' needles and 'Prime' needles have excellent points and are best used for skin surgery. Always hold the needle in the needle holder two thirds from the tip. Do not grasp the needle near the suage where the suture is attached. This part of the needle is very weak.

Suture materials

Silk has now been superseded and catgut is no longer available.

Common absorbable sutures are either braided such as Vicryl (Ethicon), Dexon (Sherwood, Davis and Geek) or monofilament such as Monocryl (Ethicon) and PDS (Ethicon). Vicryl and Dexon both retain 50% of strength at 2 to 3 weeks, Monocryl retains 50% strength at 10 days and PDS retains 50% strength at 6 weeks.

Of the many non-absorbable sutures, the most commonly used are Ethilon (polyamide) or Prolene (polypropylene). Sutures are made in various thicknesses. 6/0 is finer than 5/0, 4/0 and 3/0. 6/0 is suitable for the face; 4/0 is used on the limbs and trunk. For timing of removal of sutures see Box 12.7.

Box 12.7: Removal of sutures

Face	4–7 days
Trunk	7–10 days
Limbs	7 days

In general all monofilament surface sutures can be removed 7 days post-operatively providing adequate buried absorbable sutures have been used to hold the wound securely under tension

SURGICAL PROCEDURES

Shave biopsy/excision

- Inject the local anaesthetic subcutaneously (Figure 12.4a) and do not produce elevation of the lesion to be removed.
- Cut the lesion flat to the surrounding skin, stretching the skin firmly between the middle and forefinger of the non-dominant hand (Figure 12.4b) and pull the skin tight with the hypothenar eminence of the dominant hand.
- Begin cutting back and forth with a razor blade or surgical blade and do not stop until excision is complete (Figure 12.4c) to leave a flat surface (Figure 12.4d).
- For haemostasis, 20% aluminium chloride in 70% isopropyl alcohol is best. Driclor is an alternative. Light diathermy or cautery may be used.

Curettage

Disposable curettes are now universally available and are best.

- Hold the curette — sharp side down as you would a pencil between middle fingers, forefingers and thumb stretching the skin between the hands (Figure 12.5).
- Pull the curette gently at an angle of about 45° but firmly across the tumour from one margin to the next, separating it from the underlying skin. The action should be gentle, seeking out the plane of least resistance.
- For haemostasis, use aluminium chloride, or light diathermy or cautery.

Punch biopsy

- Mark the skin to show the preferred axis of the scar (Figure 12.6a, b).
- Stretch the skin at right angles to this.
- Rotate the punch, usually a 4 mm punch, down to its hilt. The plug will usually spring up attached to the fatty base.
- Support and lift the skin gently with a hook or forceps; do not crush the biopsy with the forceps.

231

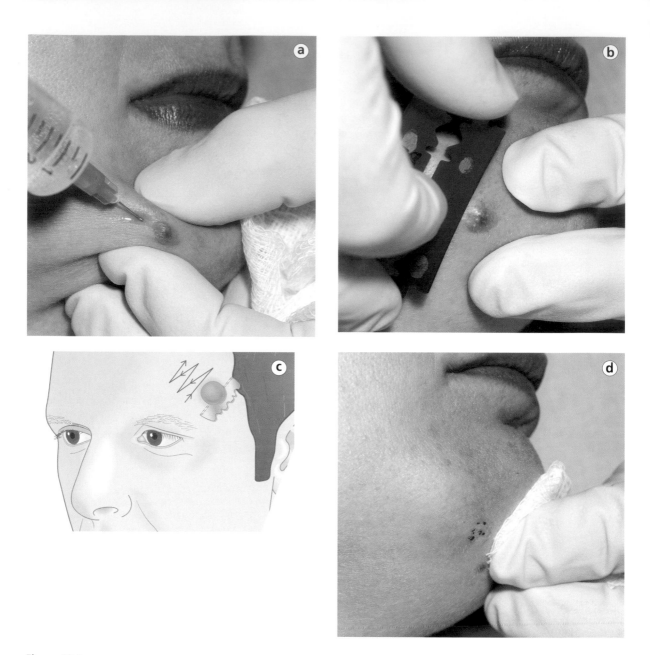

Figure 12.4
Shave biopsy. Inject (a) the local anaesthetic deeply so as not to elevate the lesion. This minimizes the risk of producing a depression in the surface. Hold the blade firmly (b) and cut continuously (c) to produce a flat defect (d).

- Cut the biopsy from its fatty base with scissors (Figure 12.6c).
- The fusiform defect (Figure 12.6d) is then easily sutured (Figure 12.6e).
- Fine 6/0 sutures on the face or 4/0 sutures on the limbs will allow faster healing and a neater scar than leaving the wound to heal by second intention.

Incisional biopsy

This is a useful technique when histological examination of the entire dermis and dermis/fat interface is needed, for example in dermal infiltrative disorders such as lymphomas, morphoea, vasculitis, panniculitis or infiltrating carcinoma (Figure 12.7).

Deep narrow wedges of the skin can be closed easily without tension. In cases of tumours, it is better to use a large 25 mm 3/8 curve needle which enters and exits wide and passes deep to the tumour. If possible avoid passing the needle point deliberately through the body of the tumour. These sutures often pull through — 'cheese wiring'.

Excision

Plan the excision carefully. *Think* beforehand of the ways the defect you will create may close. This is essential for all surgical procedures, especially on the face.

- *Scrub* the skin with antiseptic (Box 12.8).
- Using a sterile skin pen, *mark* the intended surgical excision lines around the lesion. Draw the relaxed skin tension lines in the area of the face you are working. Ask the patient to wrinkle their nose and close their eyes tightly or purse their lips to define these

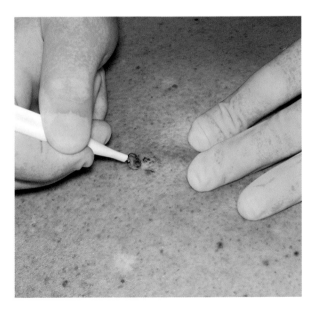

Figure 12.5
Curettage — ensure the skin is stretched firmly between the hands before curetting.

Box 12.8: Antiseptics

- Chlorhexidine 0.05% aqueous — weak antiseptic
- Chlorhexidine 0.5% spirit — better by far but allow to dry. There is a risk of fire from cautery or a diathermy spark igniting any spirit puddling in the ears or in the hair
- Povidone iodine 10% alcoholic solution — good — lets you see where you have cleaned but may obscure lines from the skin marker pen

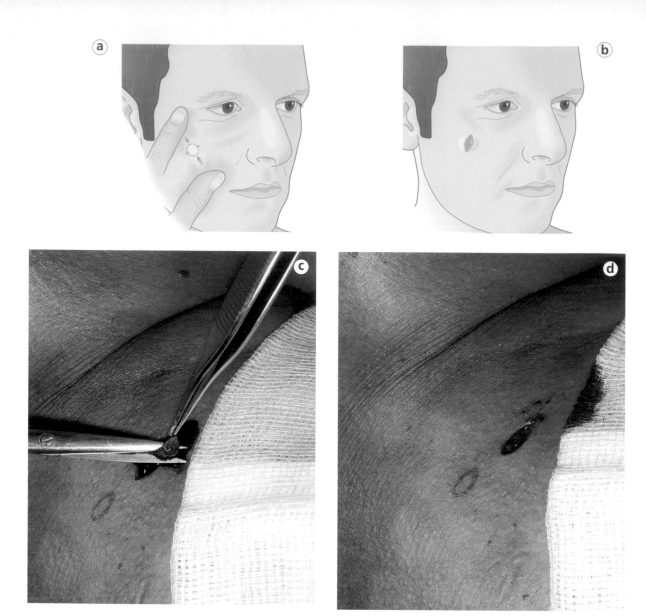

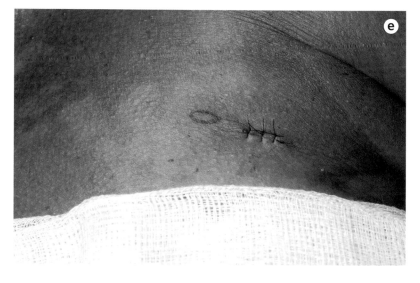

Figure 12.6
Punch biopsy — stretch the skin (a) at right angles to the intended direction of the scar (b). Remove the biopsy by cutting (c). Do not crush the specimen. The defect (d) is then sutured (e).

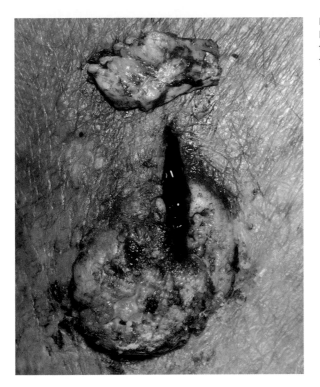

Figure 12.7
Full thickness biopsy through the edge of the tumour. This allows assessment of invasion of the tumour as far down as the fascia.

areas more clearly. This gives you information of where you would like to place the scar. Scars in wrinkle lines do not show.
- *Anaesthetize* the areas with local anaesthetic — this will cause soft tissue distortion. This is why it is essential to have drawn the skin markings beforehand.

If a fusiform excision (ellipse) is the likely outcome, the length to breadth ratio is usually 3:1. However — we seldom plan excisions as ellipses pre-operatively. It is better by far to excise the lesion first (Figure 12.8a) after debulking with the curette, and mark the upper pole of the surgical specimen with a suture and then close the defect using subcuticular sutures (Figure 12.8b) and remove the dog ears (Figures 12.8c, d) in a direction which places the scar in the optimum place (Figure 12.8e).

- *Cut* the skin perpendicular to the surface — this is much more difficult than it sounds, using your non-dominant hand and your assistant's hands to stretch and support the skin.
- *Remove the skin* carefully with curved blunt scissors with the convexity upwards. Undermine the edges — this is best done by pushing and stretching a blunt tipped scissor or needle holder to open up the plane of least resistance. This is the correct level of undermining.
- *Ensure haemostasis* is adequate using bipolar diathermy.
- *Pull* the wounds together with skin hooks and mark the skin points where the key tension-bearing subcuticular buried absorbable sutures will be placed to *close* the wound without distortion.
- *Remove the tissue protrusions* (dog ears or standing cones) in order to place the scar in the optimum position and close the surface with fine monofilament sutures (Figure 12.8e).

235

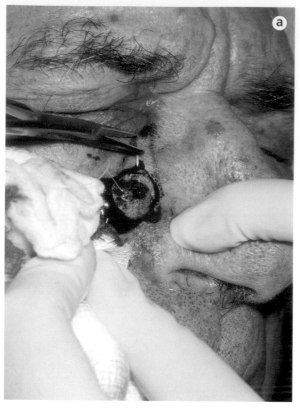

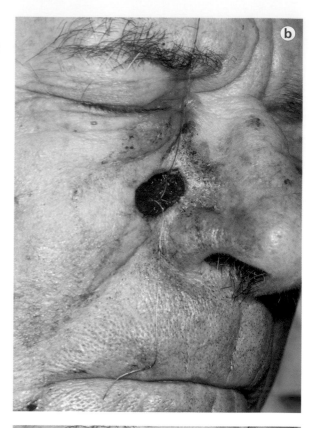

Figure 12.8
Excision of a skin tumour — excise the tumour following curettage (a) and close with subcuticular suture (b). The 'dog ears' (c) are removed (d) to place the scar in the optimum position (e).

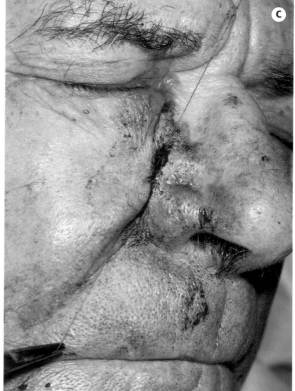

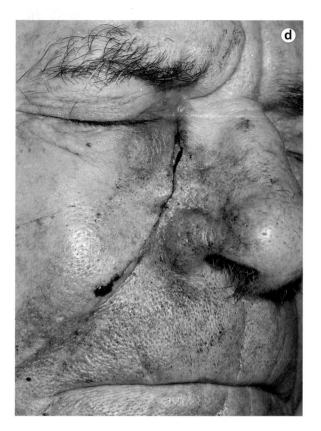 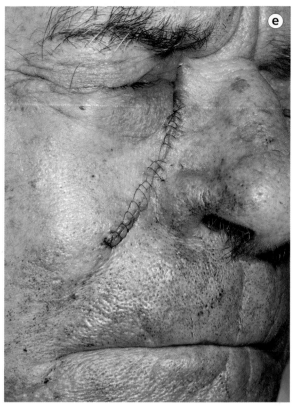

Figure 12.8 (*cont'd*)

The needle should enter and exit the wound perpendicular to the surface. This will create a slight degree of eversion which is desirable and ensures that the scar will eventually be flat and not depressed. Surface sutures will also correct the edges to the same height. Surface stitches should *not* be used as tension sutures. This is the function of the subcuticular stitches.

- *Cover* with an antiseptic gauze such as povidone iodine (Inadine) over a dressing of ointment, e.g. Polyfax. This ointment or white soft paraffin provides a lasting greasy surface to prevent the wound from drying.

Wound care

Much has been written about this — many surgeons and hospitals have their own protocol which give consistently good results. We recommend that the surface dressing should be left undisturbed and dry for 48 hours. After this time the dressing can be removed and the skin gently washed. It should be allowed to dry aided by a hairdryer if necessary but not using a towel. The sutures should then be covered with a thin film of white soft paraffin. If the wound is on the central face it can be left open; if it is on the forehead or the outer cheeks or the ears, it is best re-dressed to prevent trauma from the pillow. Obviously wounds on the trunk and limbs must be re-dressed to prevent injury and infection from clothing.

Antibiotics are not routinely prescribed except in cases where an ulcerated tumour has been excised. These tumours are frequently infected with coagulase positive *Staphylococcus aureus* and carry a risk of post-operative wound infection. There is no significant risk of bacteraemia during skin surgery and antibiotic prophylaxis for endocarditis is not required for routine dermatological procedures even in a patient with a pre-existing heart lesion.

SURGICAL TREATMENT OF MELANOMA

The treatment of primary cutaneous malignant melanoma is wide excision. Any tumour suspected as being a melanoma should be excised with a small margin of normal skin to allow histological staging. Punch biopsy, shave biopsy or curettage are not appropriate in cases of suspected melanoma. Re-excision of the scar is performed later — the margin depending on the Breslow thickness, as recommended by the BAD guidelines.[3]

Indications for sentinel node biopsy and its availability have not yet been standardized across the country.

SURGICAL TREATMENT OF NON-MELANOMA SKIN CANCER

The standard treatment is excision. Other surgical and non-surgical treatments may also be used for treatment of skin cancer and are described in the BAD guidelines.[4,5]

- For well-defined basal cell carcinomas (BCCs) up to 2 cm diameter, a 4 mm margin is necessary to excise the tumour completely in 98% of cases.[6]
- Squamous cell carcinomas (SCCs) in high risk areas such as the scalp, eyelids, ears, nose and lips and tumours with biopsy proven invasion into the subcutaneous fat will require wider margins of excision.
- Basal cell carcinomas (BCCs) occurring on the ala nasi, alar base, pre- and post-auricular area and around the inner and outer canthae may also require wider margins as these tumours often extend more widely and deeply than is clinically suspected.
- Nodular BCCs greater than 2 cm in diameter and sclerosing (morphoeic, infiltrative) BCCs and microcystic adnexal carcinoma will also require wider margins. Remember that tumour growth is *not* symmetrical around the clinical margin — larger BCCs and morphoeic BCCs are most appropriately treated with micrographic surgery.

All excised tumours must be examined histologically. The limitations of traditional histological tissue preparation for assessing adequacy of tumour excision are often not appreciated. 'Bread-loaf' cross-sectioning (Figure 12.9) permits very limited examination of the deep and lateral surgical margins.

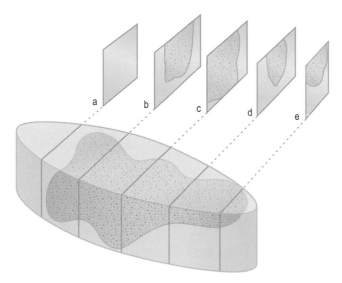

Figure 12.9
Ellipse of skin containing a tumour examined using 'bread-loaf' cross sectioning. Examination at point c and e would have demonstrated tumour invasion of the surgical margin. If sections from points a, b, and d had been examined the pathologist's report would have concluded that the tumour appears completely excised.

Complete examination of the entire surgical margin of a 1 cm specimen would require 2 500 sections — an impossible task. Typically 3 or 4 sections are prepared for the pathologist who will then examine 0.5% of the surgical margin. This explains why the pathologists often report 'tumour appears completely excised', or 'appears completely excised in the planes of the sections examined', or 'tumour does not extend to the margins of the sections examined'. As can be seen in Figure 12.9, a tumour reported as completely excised may have breached the surgical margin in areas not examined by the pathologist. Having said this, small (less than 2 cm) exophytic BCCs and SCCs excised with a 4 mm or more margin after debulking with the curette immediately prior to excision will be completely excised in nearly all cases.

THE INCOMPLETELY EXCISED TUMOUR

Over the past 35 years, several studies have reported outcomes of patients with BCCs which were reported as being incompletely excised. Recurrence rates as high as 33% at 5 years and 48% at 10 years have been reported.[7] With such high rates of 'recurrence' (which is in fact a misnomer as the tumour was never excised completely in the first place), there appears to be little justification in a 'wait and see' policy, condemning patients to long term follow up until such time as it takes the tumour to become detectable macroscopically. Some tumours reported as being incompletely excised do not subsequently recur; these sections may have been false positive margins due to incorrect embedding and orientation.

Silver staining of the tissue margins before sectioning will detect whether the histological margin seen is the true margin or not.

We teach the following approach:

- All surgical specimens should be submitted with a suture at a specified margin.
- Details of the surgical margin (in mm) should be recorded in the operative record.

- The surgical section of the specimen should be stained with silver prior to sectioning to delineate the true surgical margin.
- If the tumour is reported as incompletely excised, the surgeon and pathologist should examine the slide together to ensure that this is not a false positive margin.
- If inadequate excision has occurred, then re-excision should occur without delay. A wider and deeper excision around the scar may be adequate, otherwise there is a strong case for micrographic surgery.

MOHS' MICROGRAPHIC SURGERY

Frederick Mohs, a surgeon from Maddison, Wisconsin, USA, devised a method simple in concept to ensure complete removal of invasive BCCs. The fleshy bulk of the tumour is removed first by curettage to create a saucer shaped defect. A further margin of skin encompassing the side and base of the wound is then removed intact (Figure 12.10a) and the *surgical margin* is then prepared for horizontal sectioning. It is usual for the section to be cut into either halves or quadrants (Figure 12.10b) to permit easy tissue handling and mapping on a diagram of the anatomical site. These segments are then stained at their margins with different coloured inks.

This technique enables the entire surgical margin to be examined. If tumour is seen in these horizontal sections it *must* therefore have breached the surgical margin at that point. It is

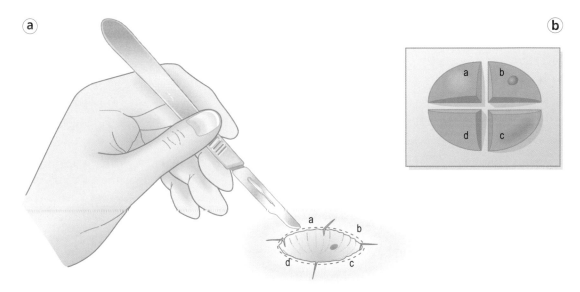

Figure 12.10
The tumour is debulked by curettage. A thin plate encompassing the entire margin and wound bed is excised (a). In this example there is residual tumour at the base of the wound. The tissue is divided into quadrants (b) and the cut edges marked with dye. The surgical margin of the tissue is sectioned horizontally to include the epidermis and deep margins in the same plane and examined under the microscope. Any tumour seen must have breached the surgical margin at this point which can be accurately located in the wound. Further specimens are removed until the surgical margins are clear of tumour.

therefore possible to identify the area in the wound bed corresponding to this point in the histological section. Further sections are then taken from this area in the wound and sectioned horizontally again to guarantee complete excision.

The technique ensures that all the tumour has been excised, yet minimizes the amount of skin removed. It is therefore tissue sparing. However, many surgeons treating basal cell carcinomas still do not completely understand the value of this technique. These doctors argue that in poorly defined tumours the simple expedient is to take a bigger margin of skin. Other surgeons claim that the use of binocular loops under bright theatre light will permit sufficiently accurate delineation of the tumour. These techniques are not good enough. It is simply not possible to see the tumour margins in a poorly delineated tumour. It is essential to understand that tumours do not invade beyond the clinical margin in a predictable way. In only one case in 300 consecutive cases of micrographically controlled excisions of BCC in our department did the tumour extend symmetrically and concentrically. Taking a wider excision margin will sacrifice more normal skin than is necessary — and the excision may still be incomplete. Remember that bread-loaf techniques are a very imperfect method of assessing tumour excision. Other popular misconceptions of micrographic surgery are that this method only just clears the tumour margin. 'Wider margins would be safer in any case.' This is not so; if the surgical margin of a tumour that grows in continuity, such as a BCC, is clear then one can be sure that the tumour has been completely excised. Tumours excised with a wider margin and then examined by bread-loaf technique will only tell the distance from the tumour to the surgical margin *in those areas where tumour is seen*. It will give no information at other areas where the tumour may have extended very close or even breached the surgical margin.

INDICATIONS FOR MICROGRAPHIC SURGERY

It is usually performed for BCCs and some SCCs, mainly on the face. It is seldom needed on the limbs and trunk where a generous margin of skin does not compromise repair.

It is primarily indicated for recurrent BCCs on the face, whatever the previous treatment — surgery, curettage, radiotherapy or cryosurgery. It is the treatment of choice for primary tumours with ill-defined margins or tumours of morphoeic type and BCCs at sites such as the inner canthus, eyelids or nose where conservation of normal tissue is paramount and where incomplete removal would have serious consequences. It is, however, a very time-consuming and therefore expensive treatment and is not therefore justified for primary treatment of small exophytic tumours.

HOW TO CLOSE SKIN DEFECTS

Following excision of any skin lesion, the resulting defect must be repaired. Several options are available (Box 12.9). Direct side to side closure is an excellent method of repair providing this does not result in any distortion.

> **Box 12.9: How to close skin defects**
>
> **Do nothing:**
>
> - laissez-faire (2nd intention)
>
> **Do something:**
>
> - primary closure
> - skin graft
> - skin flap

- It is important that skin closure does not result in tension and distortion at free margins such as the lower eyelid or the vermilion border of the lip. In such situations skin grafts or random pattern flaps may be used. A flap is a unit of skin bearing its own blood supply (the pedicle) which is moved from one location to another by advancement, rotation or transposition about a pivot point. Random pattern flaps are useful because they provide skin of good colour, texture and contour in contrast to skin grafts. Well chosen flap repairs give excellent cosmetic results and facilitate repairs not possible with other closure techniques (Figure 12.11a, b, c and d). Complications are usually a result of poor technique.
- Full thickness skin grafts are frequently used to repair defects. The donor site should be chosen which best fits the colour and texture of the recipient site. Pre- and post-auricular skin is a common donor site. For larger skin defects, skin may be taken from the supraclavicular or clavicular area. The appearance of skin grafts improves with time due to ageing.
- Wounds healing by second intention can produce excellent results, particularly on the temple, post-auricular areas and defects close to the inner canthus (Figure 12.12a, b). Second intention healing should not be used near free margins, for example, the vermilion border, alar rim, lower eyelid margin, because contraction of the wound will result in distortion.

NAIL SURGERY

Biopsy of the nail apparatus is an essential technique in dermatological surgery.[8] To perform nail surgery you will need additional instruments, nail splitters (anvil scissors) and a nail elevator — (a Freer septum elevator is an excellent alternative).

The digit must be anaesthetized by using a ring block technique. Haemostasis is important. For the finger, it is useful to apply a surgical glove to the patient's hand. The fingertip of the glove should then be snipped off and the glove rolled back to the metacarpal phalangeal joint. Alternatively a broad strip can be cut from the cuff of a surgical glove and wound round the proximal digit tightly before securing the tourniquet with artery forceps.

Avulsion of the nail

Insert the elevator under the nail pushing up against the nail plate and advance up to the lunula which represents the distal part of the matrix. Nail adhesion to the nail bed is much less at this point. Grasp the nail with a needle holder or artery forceps and twist the nail to roll it free

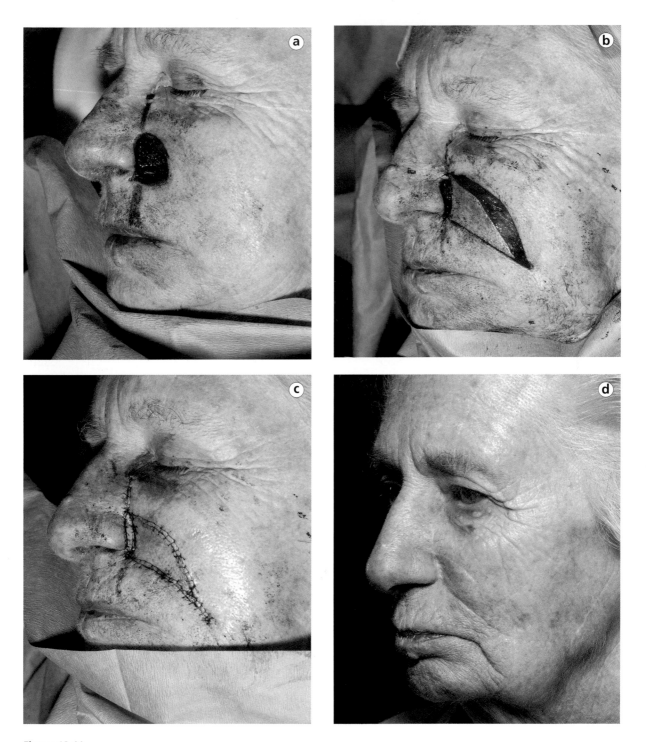

Figure 12.11
Tumour left alar base excised under micrographic control (a). Repaired with island subcutaneous pedicle flap (b). Defect on left ala repaired with small full thickness graft (c). Result 3 months later (d).

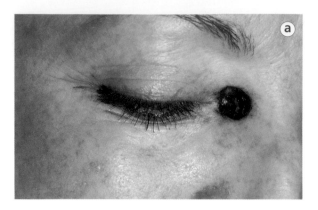
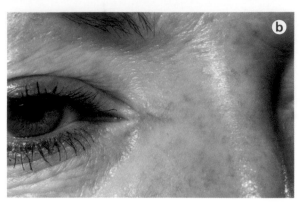

Figure 12.12 Wounds left to heal by second intention can produce excellent results. For example this defect (a), close to the inner canthus healed with an excellent cosmetic result (b).

from its attachment under the nail fold. The nail should then be pulled firmly and twisted to detach the plate from the bed using an artery forceps or needle holder. The nail bed can now be examined. Any tumour arising in the nail bed can be biopsied. If the tumour is bony hard, it is probably an exostosis and this can be confirmed with an X-ray of the distal phalanx.

Biopsy of the nail matrix and nail bed

Pigmented streaks arise usually from a melanocytic lesion in the matrix. To expose the matrix, the proximal nail fold will need to be reflected back by making incisions approximately for about 5 mm from the lateral nail fold bilaterally. The matrix should be biopsied at the origin of the pigmented streak.

For biopsies not exceeding 3 mm width, a punch biopsy will be satisfactory. If larger biopsies are needed, a horizontal (transverse) fusiform biopsy should be taken which follows the curve of the lunula. This will avoid a permanent nail defect post-operatively.

In severe nail dystrophy, the defect may arise in the bed or in the matrix. A longitudinal nail biopsy is the best investigation.

- The nail should be soaked for about 15 minutes in water before anaesthetizing the finger and applying the tourniquet.
- Using a size 11 blade, the nail plate and nail bed should be cut down to the periosteum from the free margin of the nail to a point approximately 5 mm proximal to the proximal nail fold.
- If possible, biopsy the lateral nail plate. The width of the biopsy should not exceed 3 mm.
- Remove the entire nail/nail bed/matrix with the overlying nail fold as a single unit, carefully supporting the biopsy with forceps while dissecting the tissue off the periosteum with sharp scissors.
- Orientate the specimen on a card prior to placing in the formalin fixative. Warn the pathologist beforehand or take the specimen yourself to the laboratory to ensure that the technician will embed the specimen correctly to allow the pathologists to examine the entire nail unit.

- The resulting defect should be repaired with vertical mattress sutures to ensure good approximation of the skin to the lateral nail plate.

Post-operative care

The digit will be painful for several days. Apply a non-adherent dressing over paraffin tulle. Non-steroidal anti-inflammatory drugs should be prescribed for several days. It is reasonable to prescribe antibiotics to prevent infection.

RADIOTHERAPY

This is a very effective treatment for non-melanoma skin cancer with few complications using modern dosimetry. However, the cosmetic outcome in the longer term is not always satisfactory, and is probably best avoided in younger patients. Tumour recurrence in radiotherapy scars is a problem because of high risks of poor wound healing following surgery. The same area cannot be treated twice by radiotherapy. Radiotherapy may be curative in advanced inoperable disease. Remember that radiotherapy is not cheap. Fractionated therapy will require multiple visits to the radiotherapy unit, and wound healing is slow. This can be a problem for elderly and frail patients who in fact tolerate surgery under local anaesthesia extremely well.

Radiotherapy may be useful in some patients with lentigo maligna. Cutaneous melanoma is generally radio-resistant, but it may be useful in the palliative treatment of bone and cerebral metastases.

CRYOSURGERY

Cryosurgery is the deliberate destruction of tissue by cold in a controlled manner. Various refrigerants have been used over the years — surface temperature reductions obtainable with carbon dioxide (CO_2) are $-79°C$, nitrous oxide $-75°C$ and liquid nitrogen spray $-196°C$. Most cells are killed at temperatures of -25 to $-30°C$ and this temperature can be readily achieved using liquid nitrogen spray cryosurgery.

Technique

The spray technique is most commonly used.

- The area to be treated is marked with a skin marking pen to include a margin beyond the tumour margin — the lateral freeze line.
- The spray tip (usually a 'C' spray, Cry-Ac, Brymill or less commonly a 'B' spray) is held 5 to 10 mm from the surface and liquid nitrogen is directed at the centre of the field (Figure 12.13a).
  - A visible ice field forms quickly and spreads laterally to the pre-determined margin (Figure 12.13b).

245

- The freeze time *begins* as soon as the ice ball fills the designated area.
- By slight adjustment of the flow rate and distance-to-skin, the ice field will be prevented from extending beyond the boundaries.
- The spray tip should be moved continuously over the ice field in a zig-zag or whorl pattern.[9] It is essential to establish the ice ball as quickly as possible. This ensures that the –25°C isotherm is at a deep level.
- Slow freezing produces very shallow injury. For example using a cotton bud method of delivering liquid nitrogen it is not possible to freeze colder than –18°C beyond a depth of 2 mm. 'C' sprays quickly freeze fields of 10 to 15 mm in size; 'B' spray is better used for greater areas up to 20 mm in diameter.
- Repeat freezing produces greater tissue destruction than a single freeze. Before a second freeze is given, the treated area must thaw slowly back to body temperature.
- Much cellular injury is caused by thawing. It is important to record the freeze time and the spray tip used carefully in the clinical notes.

Spray tips are now much more popular than probes. They allow greater precision. Probes are useful in confined areas such as the mouth or inside the nose.

Cryosurgery is painful. Most adults and children over 10 years of age will tolerate a single freeze up to 10 seconds. Additional lesions will usually require a local anaesthetic in children. Plain lidocaine 0.5% or 4% prilocaine should be used. Dosimetry recommended used for

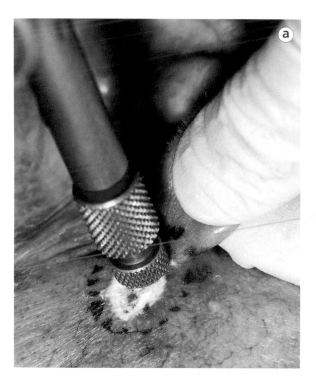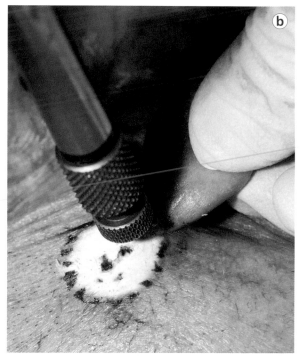

Figure 12.13
Hold the spray tip (a) 5–10 mm from the skin surface. The freeze time begins when the ice ball has filled the pre-determined area (b).

cryosurgery (Table 12.1) was established using lidocaine without adrenaline. The effects of vasoconstriction (secondary to adrenaline) on the outcomes for cryosurgery have not been critically compared to the results using plain lidocaine. At the present time it is better to use 0.5% plain lidocaine — this is much less painful in any case than any other local anaesthetic.

Liquid nitrogen spray cryosurgery can be a very effective treatment for non-melanoma skin cancer.[10] It is important to know its limitations (Box 12.10).

A note about viral warts

Cryosurgery has been used for many years for treatment of human papilloma virus infections. It works best in solitary digital or plantar viral warts. Mosaic warts on the feet are extremely resistant to cryosurgery; long freeze times up to 30 seconds are sometimes needed. This results in considerable morbidity with large blisters and swelling and discomfort necessitating wearing a soft shoe for weeks on end. Take care if contemplating treating plane warts. Treatment may result in hyper- or even hypopigmentation in people with darker complexion. Plane warts eventually will resolve without treatment leaving no marks.

Unwanted effects of cryosurgery

The patient receiving cryosurgery will have no idea of what to expect post-operatively. If treating with cryosurgery at a one-stop clinic it is essential that the patient is warned beforehand of the side effects that will occur over the following hours, days and weeks. A 5 second spray on the nose may result in a visible mark for 3 weeks. This may ruin an important social engagement; digital cryosurgery will seriously impair hand performance in

Table 12.1: Commonly used freeze time

Disease	Spray time	Lateral freeze
Digital viral warts	1×5 s; 1×10 s; 2×10 s	1 mm
Filiform warts	1×5 s	1 mm
Solitary plantar warts	1×10 s; 2×10 s	1 mm
Molluscum contagiosum	only ice formation — 'D' spray	
Seborrhoeic keratoses	1×10 s — sometimes 2×10 s	1 mm
Actinic keratoses	1×5 s; sometimes 1×10 s	1 mm
Bowen's disease	1×30 s	3 mm
Basal cell carcinoma	2×30 s	3 mm
Squamous cell carcinoma	2×30 s	3 mm
Keratoacanthoma	2×30 s	3 mm

Box 12.10: Malignant tumours not suitable for cryosurgery

- Tumours with indeterminate margins
- Tumours tethered to underlying structures
- Tumours at the alar base
- Morphoeic (infiltrating/sclerosing pattern) basal cell carcinoma
- Tumours greater than 2 cm in diameter

a person about to take a piano exam and cryosurgery on the foot will certainly stop your patient working out in the gym for several weeks.

- Immediate side effects occur in nearly all patients and include pain, swelling and blistering.
- Delayed side effects are much less predicable and are usually only seen when longer freeze-thaw cycles (30 seconds) are used. These include haemorrhage, infection (very rare) and slow healing on the lower limb. Bowen's tumour treated with a 30 second freeze or a superficial basal cell carcinoma treated with a double freeze-thaw cycle of 30 seconds on the shin or calf may take 3 to 6 months to heal. In contrast, the healing time on the face for similar conditions may be 3 to 5 weeks.
- Temporary unwanted effects are common, for example scar hypertrophy and milia. These settle without treatment.
- Impaired sensation may be noticed in the finger following digital cryosurgery and this may last for 12 to 18 months.
- Damage to hair follicles is frequently seen with longer freeze times resulting in permanent alopecia giving a poor cosmetic result.
- Melanocytes are very sensitive to cold injury and this will result in hypopigmentation and is usually permanent. It is more likely to develop after longer freeze times but slight pigment loss may be seen following short freeze cycles.

Cryosurgery should be avoided in people with type V and type VI skin.

Avoid collateral damage from splatter from the spray. For example, protect the eye using a neoprene cone or a plastic spoon if treating a lesion close to the inner or outer canthus or lower lid margin. Blue Tack may be used to protect adjacent skin if the concha of the ear is to be treated.

Liquid nitrogen is dangerous. Take care when filling the flask from the storage dewar. Spillage of nitrogen can result in cold burns. Decant the nitrogen in a large room. One volume of liquid nitrogen will release 683 times its volume of gas. Release of nitrogen causes oxygen deficiency. An atmosphere less than 18% of oxygen is hazardous.

Post-operative care following cryosurgery

The patient may take aspirin, non-steroidal anti-inflammatory drugs or paracetamol. A light non-adherent dressing gives some comfort for the first 24 hours or so. Washing the cryosurgery wound does not hinder healing. If a blister forms under much tension, it is best to burst this with a sterile needle. We treat the wounds as we manage second intention healing, namely daily lavage with water to remove any exudate and crust. The wound surface should not be left to dry, as this will increase the risk of forming a crust. A thin film of an occlusive ointment such as white soft paraffin should then be applied and covered with a non-adherent dressing.

How to stay out of trouble (Box 12.11)

Patients get cross if they develop discomfort or restriction of activity post-operatively which they were not warned about beforehand. Spend time explaining the expected side

Box 12.11: Before embarking on skin surgery involving the head and neck you should know:

- the anatomy of the superficial fascia above and below the zygomatic arch
- the surface markings of the temporal and marginal mandibular branches of the VII cranial nerve
- the surface markings of the parotid duct, and the anterior border of the masseter muscle
- the boundaries of the posterior triangle of the neck
- Erb's point

effects of all the planned treatment. Make sure the patient understands *why* they are having the test or treatment. Tell the patient what would happen if no investigation or treatment was carried out. This often convinces the patient about the need for treatment. Be certain of your diagnosis. It is very difficult to defend yourself against any action when something has gone wrong if it was not at all necessary to do the test or treatment in the first place.

Do not work under pressure or in a hurry. Accidents occur more commonly when working too fast. Do not delegate treatment to inexperienced staff who may feel reluctant to take on the job. Take care when removing epidermoid or pilar cysts on the face and neck. The deep margin of a cyst is often very close to the underlying fascia.

Remember if you fail to exercise the skill you have or claim to have you are in breach of duty of care and you are negligent. Always work within the limits of your training, ability and experience. Do not work alone. Always have an assistant to help you.

The majority of claims arising out of skin surgery result from incomplete excision of a lesion, excessive scarring, severing a nerve or other structure, post-operative infection and its sequelae, failure to obtain a histological diagnosis or failure to arrange the necessary follow-up afterwards. Make sure that all specimens are sent for histological examination and that the results are scrutinized by the clinician post-operatively.

References

1. Long CC, Motley RJ, Holt PJA. Taking the sting out of local anaesthetics. Br J Dermatol 1991; 125:452–455.
2. British Society for Dermatological Surgery Workshop Manual. Online. Available: www.bsds.org.uk
3. Roberts DLL, Anstey AV, Barlow RJ, et al. Guidelines for management of cutaneous malignant melanoma. Br J Dermatol 2002; 146:7–17.
4. Telfer NR, Colver GB, Bowers PW. Guidelines for the management of basal cell carcinoma. Br J Dermatol 1999; 141:415–423.
5. Motley RJ, Kersey P, Lawrence C. Guidelines for the management of the patient with primary cutaneous squamous cell carcinoma. Br J Dermatol 2002; 146:18–25.
6. Wolf DJ, Zitelli JA. Surgical margins for basal cell carcinoma. Arch Dermatol 1987; 123:340–344.
7. Holt PJA, Motley RJ. The treatment of basal cell carcinoma. Current Practice in Surgery 1994; 6:98–101.
8. Zook EG, Baran R, Haneke E, et al. Nail surgery and traumatic abnormalities. In: Baran R, Dawber RPR, de Berker DAR, et al, eds. Diseases of the nails and their management. 3rd edn. Oxford: Blackwell Science; 2001:425–514.
9. Dawber R, Colver G, Jackson A. Cutaneous cryosurgery. Martin Dunitz; London; 1997.
10. Holt PJA. Cryotherapy for skin cancer: results over a 5 year period using liquid nitrogen spray cryosurgery. Br J Dermatol 1988; 119:231–240.

Further reading

Eedy DJ, Breathnach SM, Walker NPJ. Surgical dermatology. Oxford: Blackwell Science; 1996.

Lawrence C. An introduction to dermatological surgery. 2nd edn. Edinburgh: Churchill Livingstone; 2002.

Laser therapy

Manjunatha Kalavala and Andrew D. Morris

INTRODUCTION

The term *laser* is an acronym for *l*ight *a*mplification by the *s*timulated *e*mission of *r*adiation. Lasers have been used in dermatology for the past four decades to treat a wide variety of conditions including vascular and pigmented lesions, tattoos, scars and unwanted hair. Cutaneous laser surgery was revolutionized by the introduction of the theory of 'Selective Photothermolysis' by Anderson and Parrish in the 1980s. The demand for laser surgery has increased substantially by patients and dermatologists alike as a result of the relative ease with which many of these lesions can be treated, combined with a low incidence of adverse post-operative sequelae. Although all of us will not be proficient in lasers, we must be well-versed in the details to be able to guide and educate our patients.

FUNDAMENTALS OF LASER THERAPY

The basic components of a laser system are the laser medium, optical cavity and pumping system (Figure 13.1). Lasers are usually named after the constituents of the laser medium. This may be a gas (e.g. argon, CO_2), a liquid (e.g rhodamine dye used in a PDL), a solid (e.g. alexandrite, diode, Er: YAG, Nd: YAG, and ruby lasers), or solid state (diode laser)

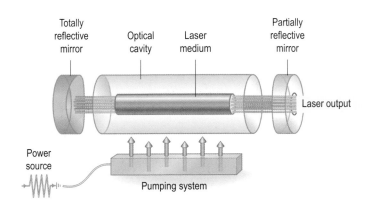

Figure 13.1
The components of a laser system.

Totally reflective mirror · Optical cavity · Laser medium · Partially reflective mirror · Laser output · Power source · Pumping system

---

Box 13.1: Abbreviations used

- APTD Argon-pumped tunable dye
- CO_2 Carbon dioxide
- CW Continuous wave
- Er: YAG Erbium: yttrium-aluminium-garnet
- Nd: YAG Neodymium: yttrium-aluminium-garnet
- KTP Potassium titanyl phosphate
- LP Long pulsed
- PDL Pulsed dye laser
- QS Quality-switched

(Box 13.1). The atoms in the laser medium are 'pumped' to an excited state by an external source of energy. This means the electrons surrounding the nucleus move from their resting orbit to an orbit of higher energy further from the nucleus. This excited state is unstable and electrons spontaneously return to their resting state and emit the absorbed energy as they do so. The energy released by this process, termed *spontaneous emission*, is emitted as light, which travels in packets of energy known as photons. When a majority of atoms in the medium are in an excited state this is termed a 'population inversion'. At this point the photons will travel along the long axis of the cavity and are increasingly likely to collide with atoms which are in an excited state. *Stimulated emission* occurs when an electron in an already excited state absorbs a photon of light and emits *two* photons of light while returning to the resting state orbit. Stimulated photons have identical wavelength and frequency. Reflecting mirrors are placed on either end of the cavity so that light travels back and forth within the cavity promoting further amplification. One of the mirrors is only partially reflective allowing a small portion of the light to travel out of the cavity as laser light, through a delivery system for transmission to the operator hand piece. Delivery systems may take the form of a fibre optic cable or articulated arms.

PROPERTIES OF LASER LIGHT

Monochromaticity

Laser light is of a single discrete wavelength determined by the laser medium. Cutaneous lesions contain targets or *chromophores* such as water, melanin, haemoglobin or tattoo ink. Chromophores can be specifically targeted by laser light of certain wavelengths (Figure 13.2).

Coherence

The waves are in phase in time and space.

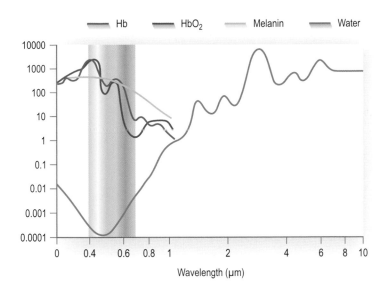

Figure 13.2
Absorption spectra of principal cutaneous chromophores.

Collimation

Laser light is a narrow, intense beam of light capable of propagation across long distances without divergence. Collimated light can be focused into small spot sizes allowing for precise tissue destruction.

SELECTIVE PHOTOTHERMOLYSIS

When laser is used on the skin, the light may be absorbed, reflected, transmitted or scattered (Figure 13.3). Light must be absorbed by tissue for a clinical effect to take place. Once laser energy is absorbed in the skin, three basic effects are possible: photothermal, photochemical, or photomechanical.

- *Photothermal effect* occurs when a chromophore absorbs the corresponding wavelength of energy and destruction of the target results from the conversion of the absorbed energy to heat.
- *Photochemical effects* derive from native or photosensitizer related reactions that serve as the basis of photodynamic therapy (PDT).
- Extremely rapid thermal expansion can lead to acoustic waves and subsequent *photomechanical destruction* of the absorbing tissue.

Photothermal and photomechanical reactions are most commonly observed in current cutaneous laser surgery practice.

Our understanding of laser-tissue interaction was greatly enhanced with Anderson and Parrish's *theory of selective photothermolysis*. The theory describes how controlled destruction of a targeted lesion is possible without significant thermal damage to surrounding normal tissue. Definition of key terms is given in Box 13.2. To achieve selective photothermolysis,

Figure 13.3
Laser-tissue interactions.

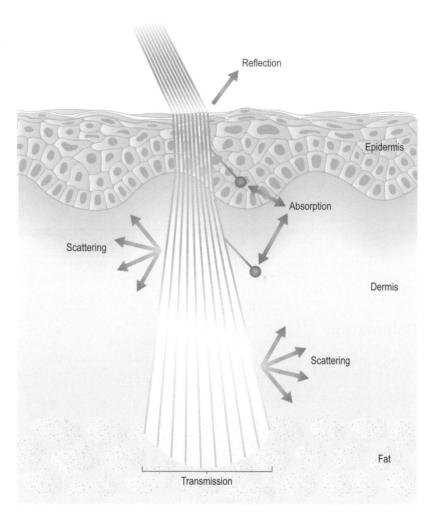

Reflection

Epidermis

Absorption

Scattering

Dermis

Scattering

Fat

Transmission

Box 13.2: Definition of key terms

- *Pulse duration:* exposure duration of the tissue to light
- *Thermal relaxation time:* time required for the targeted site to cool to one half of its peak temperature immediately after laser irradiation
- *Fluence:* energy absorbed by target tissue in joules/cm²

---

a suitable *wavelength* preferentially absorbed by the target tissue or chromophore is selected. To minimize thermal injury to surrounding structures, the laser *pulse duration* should be equal to or shorter than the thermal relaxation time of the intended target. *Fluence* must be sufficient to achieve destruction of the target within the allotted time. Therefore laser parameters (wavelength, pulse duration and fluence) can be tailored for specific cutaneous applications to effect maximal target destruction with minimal collateral thermal damage.

Consideration must also be given to the depth of target structure. In general, the depth of penetration of laser energy increases with wavelength.

Lasers are also classified according to the *pulse characteristics* of the beam (Box 13.3). Pulsed and quasi-CW systems are better adapted for cutaneous laser surgery on the basis of the principles of selective photothermolysis because the thermal relaxation time of most cutaneous chromophores is very short. The pulse width is varied so that it approximates the thermal relaxation time of the chromophore.

Cooling

By cooling the epidermis, higher fluences and therefore higher temperature elevations are possible in the targeted structures in the dermis while preserving the epidermis, particularly important in pigmented skin. Almost all cooling strategies will provide some pain relief. Cooling can be before the laser pulse (pre), during the pulse (parallel), or after the pulse (post). Cooling methods include:

- Contact cooling precooling with an aluminium roller, ice or gold gels, chilled sapphire window cooled to 4°C, copper plate.
- Cold air.
- Cryogen spray cooling.

Anaesthesia

Most laser procedures are associated with some discomfort. The sensations described range from mild warmth, to 'the snap of a rubber band' or 'bacon grease spatter', to severe burning pain. In many cases, topical anaesthetic preparations like EMLA or Ametop alleviate most of the discomfort. For more invasive treatments, the pain can be quite intense, necessitating the use of anaesthetics, analgesics and/or anxiolytics.

Laser safety

- *Eye protection:* Laser light can cause permanent retinal damage and vision loss. Eye protection in the form of optically coated glasses or goggles for the specific laser being used is required for all persons present in the room during laser treatment. If the goggles obstruct the treatment area in the periorbital area, use of an anodized external metal eye cup can be used to protect the patient's eyes. If the eyelids are to be treated, a metal corneal eye shield should be placed on the eye using topical anaesthesia to protect the

---

Box 13.3: Laser classification

- *CW lasers:* emit a constant beam of light, e.g. CO_2 laser
- *Quasi-CW laser:* pulses at very rapid rates and low energy with very short rest times between pulses with almost continuous waves, e.g. KTP, copper vapour
- *Pulsed laser systems:* emit high-energy laser light in ultra short pulse durations
  - *Long pulsed:* pulse durations of 450 microseconds to 40 milliseconds, e.g. PDL
  - *Very short pulsed:* pulse durations of 5–100 nano seconds, e.g. QS ruby, alexandrite, Nd:YAG
  - *Super pulsed:* produce very short pulses in a repetitive pattern, e.g. modified CO_2 lasers

globe. The door to the treatment room must be kept closed and locked with an external warning sign during laser firing to protect innocent intruders or passers-by from possible injury.

- *Accidental fires* can occur in the presence of circulating oxygen, ignition of surgical tubing, sponges, drop clothes or drapes. To minimize these risks, oxygen, if present, should be minimized; saline soaked drapes or clothes should be used intra-operatively; exposed hair-bearing areas should be kept moist; and alcohol-based skin preparations should be strictly avoided. In addition, lasers should be kept in the standby mode when not in use to avoid inadvertent firing.
- *Electrical hazards* can be eliminated by dedicating a specific electric outlet for each laser and by avoiding the use of extension cords.
- *Infection risk:* smoke and aerosolized fragments have been reported to contain human papilloma virus, HIV p24 antigen, other viruses and cellular materials. A smoke evacuator with clean filters and tubing minimizes infection risk when using ablative lasers.

PATIENT SELECTION AND COUNSELLING

- The patient should be informed about all aspects of the procedure as well as the risks and benefits of the procedure and written consent should be obtained before the procedure. In general, side effects and complications include vesiculation, crusting, pigmentation abnormalities (hyperpigmentation and hypopigmentation) and scarring. Treatment of vascular lesions may result in a variable degree of short-term purpura.
- Pre-operative laser evaluation should include a basic medical history including documentation of medications and allergies. A history of abnormal scarring, excessive sun exposure, allergic or inflammatory conditions, herpes simplex virus outbreaks, immune disorders, or cosmetic procedures within the involved area should also be ascertained.
- Ensure that the patient is not recently tanned. This is important because epidermal melanin may interfere with laser treatment and increase the risks of scarring, hypo- or hyperpigmentation.
- Patients who have been on oral retinoids within the previous 12 months have increased risk of scar formation and poor healing.
- Oral antiviral prophylaxis should always be considered for patients with a history of herpes simplex (HSV) infections undergoing ablative laser treatment. If active HSV infection is present on the day of laser treatment, the appointment should be cancelled and delayed until the area has healed completely. The patient can be placed on appropriate pre-operative prophylactic antiviral therapy prior to initiation of therapy.
- Obtain photographs at baseline and at regular intervals to monitor progress.
- It is important for patients to understand the importance of good wound care after a laser procedure. Written post-operative instructions should be provided.

PRACTICAL POINTS (Box 13.4)

To learn how to operate a laser system can be a daunting task for the beginner. Read the user's manual and familiarize yourself with the machine. Work with experienced laser operators and attend a laser training course.

CUTANEOUS APPLICATIONS OF LASER THERAPY

Laser systems currently available and their cutaneous applications are listed in Table 13.1. In a single centre, all lasers may not be available and it is important to know the strengths and limitations of available laser systems. Treatment of some common skin conditions is discussed briefly.

Treatment of vascular lesions

Cutaneous vascular lesions are one of the most common indications for laser treatment in dermatology. The target chromophore in the treatment of vascular lesions is oxyhaemoglobin. The peaks of oxyhaemoglobin absorption are at 418 nm, 542 nm and 577 nm. Pulsed dye lasers are the laser of choice for most congenital and acquired vascular lesions because of their superior clinical efficacy and low risk profile. PDL treatments are performed with fluences ranging from 3–10 J/cm^2 and a spot size of 2–10 mm with no more than 10% overlap. Other laser and light systems that are currently used to treat vascular lesions include the intense pulsed light, KTP, diode, alexandrite and Nd: YAG lasers.

Box 13.4: Practical points

- Perform laser test spots in all patients prior to treating an entire lesion to determine the treatment parameters
- To establish initial parameters, read the user's manual and consult experienced laser surgeons who have been working with the laser being used
- Begin with the lowest energy fluence. At subsequent treatments fluence can be increased by small increments of 0.5 to 1 joule as necessary. Remember, using too high an energy fluence can result in thermal injury and scarring
- Position the laser hand piece at a 90 degree angle perpendicular to the skin surface
- Ensure that the hand piece is held at the appropriate distance from the patient
- Try to deliver the pulses close to one another without significant overlap. While a small amount of overlap will generally not have an adverse effect, repeatedly delivering multiple pulses to the same area can result in unwanted thermal injury and scarring
- In darker-skinned patients, lasers having longer wavelengths are generally safer as they spare injury to the epidermis to a greater degree than shorter wavelength lasers

Table 13.1: Cutaneous application of lasers

Laser type	Wavelength (nm)	Cutaneous application
Argon	488/514	vascular lesions
APTD	577/585	vascular lesions
Copper vapour/bromide	510/578	pigmented lesions, vascular lesions
KTP	532	pigmented lesions, vascular lesions
Nd: YAG	frequency doubled 532	pigmented lesions, red/orange/yellow tattoos
PDL	510	pigmented lesions
	585/595	vascular lesions, hypertrophic/keloid scars, striae, verrucae, nonablative dermal remodelling
Ruby	694	QS: pigmented lesions, blue/black/green tattoos normal mode: hair removal
Alexandrite	755	QS: pigmented lesions, blue/black tattoos normal mode: hair removal, leg veins
Diode	800–810	hair removal, leg veins
Nd: YAG	1064	QS: pigmented lesions, blue/black/green tattoos normal mode: hair removal, leg veins, nonablative dermal remodelling
Nd: YAG	long-pulsed 1320	nonablative dermal remodelling
Diode	long-pulsed 1450	nonablative dermal remodelling, acne
Er: glass	1540	nonablative dermal remodelling
Er: YAG (pulsed)	2490	ablative skin resurfacing, epidermal lesions
CO_2 (CW)	10 600	actinic cheilitis, verrucae, rhinophyma
CO_2 (pulsed)	10 600	ablative skin resurfacing, epidermal/dermal lesions
Intense pulsed light source (IPL)	515–1200	superficial pigmented lesions, vascular lesions, hair removal, nonablative dermal remodelling

Treatment of pigmented lesions and tattoos

The majority of benign epidermal and dermal pigmented lesions respond to high-energy QS red and infrared lasers, although the response is variable. The chromophore is melanin. Superficially located pigment is best treated with shorter wavelength lasers (eg. 532 nm QS Nd: YAG). For removal of deeper pigment longer wavelength lasers are needed (e.g. 755 nm alexandrite, 1064 nm QS Nd: YAG). The treatment of melanocytic naevi is controversial. Treatment should only be undertaken if there is no doubt about the nature of the lesion. The main concerns in treating melanocytic naevi with lasers are the possibility that this may increase the risk of future malignant transformation (there is no evidence to support this at the present time) and that any future malignant change (whether related to laser treatment or not) could be masked, leading to a diagnostic delay.

In tattoo removal, the target chromophores are small particles of tattoo ink within macrophages or scattered extracellularly throughout the dermis. For optimal pigment removal, the choice of laser is based on the absorption spectra of the ink colours present within the tattoo. Black pigments are best treated with QS alexandrite (755 nm) or QS Nd: YAG (1064 nm). Blue and green inks respond well to alexandrite laser. Red, yellow and orange inks respond well to 532 nm QS Nd: YAG laser. In general, professional tattoos are more difficult to treat than amateur tattoos.

Treatment of hypertrophic scars, keloids and striae

PDL has been shown to produce striking improvement in scar erythema, pliability, bulk and dysaesthesia. Significant clinical improvement in hypertrophic scars is usually noted after 1 or 2 treatments. Keloids and very thick or proliferative hypertrophic scars may require additional laser treatments or simultaneous use of intralesional corticosteroid or 5-fluorouracil injections. Significant clinical improvement of early erythematous striae can be achieved using low fluence PDL irradiation. However, only minimal to modest effects are observed in mature striae.

Laser photoepilation

Lasers and IPL sources with wavelengths in the red or near-infrared region (600–1200 nm) effectively target melanin within the hair shaft, hair follicle epithelium and heavily pigmented matrix. LP ruby (694 nm), LP alexandrite (755 nm), pulsed diode (800 nm), QS and LP Nd: YAG (1064 nm) and IPL (590–1200 nm) sources are currently used for laser photoepilation.

Cutaneous laser resurfacing

Ablative laser systems such as pulsed CO_2 and erbium:YAG lasers are used in laser resurfacing of severely photodamaged facial skin, photoinduced facial rhytides, dyschromias and atrophic scars.

Eradication of benign, premalignant and malignant lesions can also be achieved with ablative laser systems. Benign lesions such as seborrhoeic keratoses, verrucae vulgaris, xanthelasma, sebaceous gland hyperplasia, syringomata and trichoepithelioma can be successfully treated. Treatment of premalignant and malignant skin lesions, including actinic cheilitis, superficial basal cell carcinoma and Bowen's disease has been reported.

Ablative laser resurfacing is associated with significant morbidity until complete re-epithelialization occurs.

Nonablative laser systems in the infrared portion of the electromagnetic spectrum (1000–1500 nm) create a dermal wound without disruption of the epidermis. Nonablative laser resurfacing has the advantage of producing virtually no external wound.

CONCLUSION

Lasers have essentially revolutionized cosmetic dermatology and have provided safe and reliable means for treating a wide variety of cutaneous pathologies. Laser surgery is constantly evolving with technological innovations. It is essential to keep ourselves updated with this everexpanding specialty.

Further reading

Lanigan SW. Lasers in dermatology.: London; Springer-Verlag; 2000.

Goldberg D. Lasers and lights: vascular, pigmentation, scars, medical applications (Procedures in cosmetic dermatology series). WB Saunders; 2005.

Dover JS. Illustrated cutaneous and aesthetic laser surgey. : Stamford, CA: Appleton and Lange; 1999.

Index